The Gluten-Free Cheat Sheet

THE
Gluten-Free
Cheat Sheet

• Go G-Free in 30 Days or Less •

APRIL PEVETEAUX

A PERIGEE BOOK

A PERIGEE BOOK
Published by the Penguin Group
Penguin Group (USA) LLC
375 Hudson Street, New York, New York 10014

USA • Canada • UK • Ireland • Australia • New Zealand • India • South Africa • China

penguin.com

A Penguin Random House Company

THE GLUTEN-FREE CHEAT SHEET

ISBN: 978-0-399-17299-1

This book has been registered with the Library of Congress.

First edition: July 2015

PRINTED IN THE UNITED STATES OF AMERICA

10 9 8 7 6 5 4 3 2 1

Text design by Kristin del Rosario

For my adorable—yet brutal—taste testers,
Esmé, Judah, and Aaron

·CONTENTS·

Hi there. My name is April, and I would like to apologize to you for having to pick up this book. Because if you're even thinking about going gluten-free, you're probably pretty sad right now, and for that I offer my most sincere condolences. Because croissants. If you are here because someone has told you, or you've discovered on your own, that gluten should be banished from your diet, you may be wondering how to start this new life without wheat, barley, rye, and triticale. (You're also wondering what the heck triticale is, right?) You're probably looking for some guidance, someone to scream with (or at), and a killer recipe for gluten-free cake. My gluten-intolerant friend, you have come to the right place.

In 2010, I began having incredibly unpleasant gastro-intestinal "distress." I think you get where I'm going with that. I had unexplained eczema that did not go away with traditional treatment, had joint pain that was fit for a ninety-year-old, and lost a dramatic amount of weight. It started slowly, then amped up by the end of the year, during the month I tried to be a vegetarian. Yes, I did consume a ton of pasta, and yes, that helped to really kick things into gear. After being violently ill for three months straight, I was diagnosed with celiac disease in January 2011, thanks to a super-sharp gastro-enterologist who sent me for an endoscopy (the gold standard for celiac diagnosis). The diagnosis was quickly and positively confirmed, and I was in for an extreme lifestyle change, or risk even more illness. Naturally, I jumped in with both feet, because no pastry is worth ruining your life.

Having never heard of gluten, celiac, or "cross-contamination," I was in for a huge learning curve as I navigated this new, and unpleasant, state of being. As a writer and an editor, I headed right to the bookstore and online to learn as much as I possibly could about what I was being forced into. The news was not great. At the same time, I was struck by the ridiculousness of having a disease that is activated by a sandwich. I was pretty sure I wasn't alone out there in wondering what the heck was up with gluten, and so I started my blog, Gluten Is My Bitch. After experimenting with gluten-free flours, throwing myself on the mercy of waiters and chefs all over the country, and complaining end-lessly about the lack of donuts in my life, I found my groove and my audience. It turns out that a lot of you out there are just as irritated about this forced diet and are also wondering where all the good gluten-free do-nuts are actually hiding.

I decided to dig in even more by writing my first book, Gluten Is My Bitch: Rants, Recipes, and Ridiculous-

ness for the Gluten-Free, and voilà! Here I am today to continue educating about gluten-free living and providing you with delicious recipes to make you happy no matter how sad you are about pizza.

I've been there (actually, I'm still there and will continue to be there for the rest of my life), and I'm here to tell you that you will get through this time of soft pretzel deprivation and come out on the other side feeling healthier, happier (that is, until you find yourself walking by a pizzeria), and more well adjusted, digestion-wise. Will there be rough times? Oh yes, there will be. (See smells of pizzeria, two sentences ago.) Will there be times when you take the word "quinoa" in vain? You bet. But there will also be many delicious meals, fun travels, and new food discoveries as you change your diet, which was probably overloaded with donuts anyway. Or perhaps that's just me.

If you're exploring the idea of a gluten-free diet, or are being forced into going on a gluten-free diet, there are tricks and tips that will make this journey a heck of a lot easier. One might even say there are "cheats." Hence, the title of this book. After living with, writing about, and complaining to friends and loved ones about the gluten-free diet, I've got some pretty great solutions to those moments of "You mean I can't eat that either?" And I'm committed to empowering the gluten-free; which is why I can't wait to teach everyone how to eat, live, and survive this dramatic lifestyle and/or medical change. It's easy! Okay, it's totally not easy, but with my tips, recipes, coaching, and regular rounds of cursing and punching the couch pillows, WE CAN DO IT.

Wait, why do we want to do it?

That's an excellent question. You may have just received a celiac disease diagnosis or another autoimmune disease diagnosis that requires a gluten-free diet. Or you may have just realized that every time you eat at the Olive Garden, you find the unlimited breadsticks to be more of a problem than a bonus. Some of you just feel better when you go gluten-free even without a diagnosis of celiac disease, intolerance, sensitivity, or any medical reason—and you're welcome here, too. Now, for those of you who were given this book by a concerned relative, or a friend who swears going gluten-free changed her life, or (more embarrassingly) a roommate/coworker/spouse who thinks you need to change your diet for, umm, odiferous reasons, I'm going to help you understand the weird world of the gluten-free diet as well. Maybe you'll join us, or maybe you'll ignore us and go back to your brioche-eating ways. Either way, read on! You'll certainly have more of a handle on dining out in mixed company and perhaps some sympathy for those of us who have no choice in the matter of diet. I mean, this whole gluten-free diet fad has to be popular for some reason, right? It's popular because people outside the celiac disease and gluten-intolerant community have found some kind of benefit to going gluten-free. Maybe that will be you.

For those of us who have no choice in the matter, it's a fact that gluten does wreak havoc on the digestive system, the immune system, and the mood. I'm not sure how something so delicious can be so problematic. I'm really not. But I'm here to tell you that no matter why you're going gluten-free, it's going to be okay. Guess what? It's totally going to be okay.

They say unhealthy patterns can be broken in something like 28 days. But we're talking about gluten here: the delicious protein that helps croissants be flaky, donuts be airy, and baguettes be filled with holes and goodness. I say you need 30 days to get over the shock to your brand-new gluten-free system. Also, a 30-day plan is so much better because you can be all, "I made it a month! I can do eleven more!" Or you can say, "I did this for an entire month, and I see no reason to go on." Really, it's your gluten-free choice. (Again, unless you have celiac disease, in which case there's no choice unless you consider chronic illness and potential death as a "choice" equal to skipping burrito night. Which you don't, right?)

But if you are one of the more than 20 million Americans who have celiac disease, gluten sensitivity, a wheat allergy, or another autoimmune disease that requires you to get rid of gluten, you're going to need a hand so you can stay healthy. I won't lie: It's going to be a dramatic shift in your day-to-day life as well as your long-term goals (can you say, finding a safe vacation spot?). But if you can replace that gluten craving with delicious food that will not kill you, well, that's awesome, right?

Which is exactly what this book will help you do. I've gone through the various stages of gluten grief and come out the other side with a heck of a lot of fantastic ideas and recipes to make me forget about my gluten-free woes. With my new attitude and arsenal of gluten-free helpers, I will take you on a journey for the next 30 days filled with many tears, much laughter, and SO MUCH HIGH-FIVING. I'm here; you're here; let's talk about how we're going to make this gluten-free living thing happen.

First, I'll break the news gently about all those problems with gluten, and then I'll play a violin as I start tossing the delicious gluten food out of your pantry, but *then* I'm going to whip up some flavorful, melt-in-your-mouth gluten-free meals to make you happier than a pig in a truffle patch. Or a foodie in a truffle patch. Take your pick.

By the end of this 30-day journey, you will have 100 new gluten-free recipes in your repertoire. Easy and delicious ones, in fact.

You may be wondering who I am to make such claims. Well, I was you. After my celiac disease diagnosis in 2011, I also raged against the bread machine. I did not know how Saturday mornings would ever bring me joy again until, that is, I discovered the beauty of gluten-free waffles. (The dirty little secret of the gluten-free is that pancakes and waffles are not discernible with or without gluten. WIN.) I worked my way back from avoiding bistros for fear of the smell of a baguette to marching right up to the maître d' and having a frank conversation about steak frites. I am the girl who now knows how to make a gluten-free biscuit with gluten-free gravy and—of course—sausage. (Yes, I am also the girl who was raised in Oklahoma.) The point is, I freaked out when I was told to cut gluten out of my diet, but now I'm a functional gluten-free member of society who is still able to have a good time at any given holiday party. And you can be, too.

Most important, I'm the girl who cooks every night I'm not out on the town, and have been doing so since getting my diagnosis back in 2011. My 100 recipes consist mostly of meals my family and I enjoy on a regular basis, and you and your family can adopt them as your own. Sometimes we enjoy tacos, other times we go Paleo, and we especially love vegetables, so there's really something for everyone. What this means is that I have some foolproof recipes for you, which you can make any night of the week. I also have some fancy stuff for those times you need to impress the people who don't think you can eat well without white flour. But let's be honest: We mostly need to know how to make dinner after a hard day at the office—a meal that's quick, easy, and satisfying.

So let's talk gluten and why we're giving it up. Then let's move on to the baked Brie and gluten-free cocktails, shall we? *Salut!*

ONE

The Problem with Gluten

Who, What, and Why

· · · · · · · ·

When someone first talks to you about removing gluten from your diet, you'll certainly feel a pain in the breadbasket. But once you stand up straight and take a breath, you're going to wonder what, exactly, gluten is anyway. In fact, many people have shown via late-night television that they really don't know what it is they're no longer eating. I want to make sure you are not one of those people. Especially if you happen to dine out where I do because, wow, NOT COOL.

There are multiple ways a body can react to gluten. The three most common medical reasons to go gluten-free include (1) celiac disease, (2) non-celiac gluten sensitivity, or (3) a wheat allergy. While all three of these conditions are very different, they all have the same solution—remove gluten from the diet. Or in the case of the wheat allergy, just remove the wheat and go crazy with triticale, rye, and barley.

Meet the Celiacs

Celiac disease is an autoimmune disorder, which means your body's immune system believes it has been compromised and begins to fight off invaders. When you're a celiac, gluten is that invader. And that invader is as brutal as Vlad the Impaler. For a celiac, like me, gluten comes into my body and my body says, "No way." Then my body freaks out and all sorts of horrible things start happening that, if left alone to do their thing, could lead to death. Yep, it's that serious. Even though we may look okay on the outside, those of us with celiac are completely torn up on the inside. Suddenly your body is attacking itself, ripping out those poor defenseless villi in your small intestine and making you sick as a very sick dog. A sampling of celiac symptoms includes incredibly unpleasant gastrointestinal distress, peeling skin, and joints on fire. But really, there are so many ways gluten can hurt a body.

It is estimated that 1 in 100 people have the autoimmune disease of celiac, but many remain undiagnosed.[1] In fact, at the time of this publication, the estimate is that there are 2.5 million Americans who remain undiagnosed with celiac and are experiencing damage to their bodies by not following a gluten-free diet. According to Dr. Alessio Fasano in his book *Gluten Freedom*, it wasn't until the past decade that physicians believed that celiac disease even existed in the United States. Hence, the explosion of new celiac disease diagnoses in North America and the popularity of the gluten-free diet. For many people in the United States with celiac

---

[1] Celiac Disease Foundation, 2014, celiac.org.

disease, this recent discovery meant years and years of suffering before a doctor was willing and able to get to the bottom of gastrointestinal, skin, and a load of other problems. So when people ask you, "Why is everyone gluten-free all of a sudden?" you can answer, "Because no one knew what celiac disease was in America until 2003," and put an end to the idea that those of us who don't eat gluten are just trying to be trendy.

They Simply Won't Tolerate It

There are even more of you out there who don't have an "official" celiac diagnosis (and therefore are also lacking the torn-up villi, lucky dogs) but suffer greatly when you ingest gluten. You are the gluten intolerants, or you have a gluten sensitivity, depending on who's telling the story. And there are a lot of you in this category—in fact, six times the number of those of us with a celiac disease diagnosis. There are 18 million people with a gluten sensitivity in America who don't have the "official" celiac diagnosis but experience the same symptoms.[2] The only good thing about having this diagnosis vs. celiac is that your villi will remain intact, and you won't have to worry about a lack of absorption of vitamins and minerals in your diet as a result. But it is equally unpleasant in every other way. All of you out there who have gluten sensitivity or are gluten intolerant may have a hard time being taken seriously, but your pain is similar to or worse than celiac disease sufferers depending on your symptoms.

---

[2] National Foundation of Celiac Awareness, 2014, celiaccentral.org.

Ahhhh-Choo!

The wheat allergy crew are very different from these other two, although it's possible to have a wheat allergy *and* celiac (and I know from experience). But if you're battling a wheat allergy on its own, your symptoms will be different. Wheat is one of the top eight food allergens in America, so it's not that unusual a diagnosis either. Your wheat allergy symptoms will look more like other food allergy symptoms, which can range from itchiness and swelling to the incredibly frightening anaphylaxis, which is immediately life threatening. Depending on the severity of your symptoms, you may have an easier, or a much more difficult, time keeping your diet safe from a gluten invasion. If you do have a wheat allergy, you should ask your doctor for an EpiPen to carry around with you in case you do accidentally ingest gluten, and make sure you know how to use it. If you do have to engage your EpiPen, have someone take you to the emergency room immediately following the injection to receive treatment.

The Randoms

Those of you who have other autoimmune diseases, such as rheumatoid arthritis, lupus, gluten ataxia, or Crohn's disease, may also feel a million times better once gluten is cut out of your diet (and in the case of gluten ataxia, you *must* be on a gluten-free diet). And here's a shout-out to all of you supposed IBS sufferers who have realized that maybe that IBS diagnosis was not all that, and it is, in fact, gluten that makes everything go all "IBS."

All of this is to say that gluten can be very, very, very

bad for a select group of people. Or it could simply make your stomach swell up and ruin your evening. There is definitely a wide range of gluten reactions on the spectrum. This is why there are two schools of thought on whether all of us should describe our gluten condition as an allergy when we have to explain our dining restrictions to a waiter or someone else preparing our food. Since "allergy" sounds so severe and dramatic, the people preparing your meal realize that care must be taken with your food. Some people feel that is not really fair if we are not, in fact, in danger of dropping dead at the table. After all, you're telling a stranger that your life is in her hands. But it's also why those of us who have celiac or an intolerance use the word sometimes, so we *will* be taken seriously. Sometimes you have to go for comprehension over accuracy when it could mean the difference between a great meal and winding up sick in bed for weeks.

One Gluten Story

When anyone, regardless of diagnosis, reacts negatively to gluten, it can be pretty horrible. Having a reaction to gluten messes up your life in so many disgusting, painful, annoying ways. Before my diagnosis and removal of gluten from my diet, I had the pleasure of experiencing what I thought was eczema all over my face, diarrhea multiple times a day, and joints that felt like they would break if I moved. Plus, I would pass out whenever I sat down. Just from eating gluten. I had a preschooler and a tiny baby when the problems started, and I can tell you with great authority: It's not so easy to take care of little kids when you're living in the bathroom and/or the bed.

This is why I work so hard to avoid gluten today, because that same exact thing happens to me if someone slips me some soy sauce in a dressing, or flour in my queso (which should *never* happen—NEVER). My life is disrupted, my children don't get their mother, and my work does not get done. Add to those good times that every time gluten enters my body I'm upping my chances of osteoporosis, cancer, stroke, and a host of other good-time diseases, and I'm pretty dang motivated not to eat gluten. Do I want a Krispy Kreme? Absolutely. But being knocked out for weeks at a time, and really having to soldier on due to work and life commitments, makes that sugary glaze not worth the pain.

Gluten makes us very, very sick. And while you can't always see the results standing in front of you, it's not only there but painful. Getting gluten-ed is no joke, even though some comedians try to make it into one. I wouldn't wish gluten intolerance, celiac, or any other food issue on my worst enemy—no matter how trendy. Having an adverse reaction to food is physical, not psychological (well, except for the depression and anxiety, which are other side effects), and not at all funny (even if I do joke about it at my own expense from time to time).

So Gluten Is Horrible . . . but What Is It?

So now you know that gluten can really mess up a certain percentage of the population. But what the heck is it? The scientifically accurate description of gluten is as follows: Gluten consists of the two proteins that exist in wheat, barley, rye, and triticale. These two groups of proteins are called gliadins and glutenins. Sure that glutenin gang sounds the worst, but it's much more complicated than that. The peptides in gliadins are the harmful guys. (And honestly, the glutenins peptides could be as well; we just KNOW the gliadin gang is pretty horrible.) They like to attack the small intestine, which sets off a whole set of problems. Rather than me pretending to be a scientist, let me just explain what's shaking with gluten in the most basic terms—the terms you, as a gluten avoider, need to know, and nothing more.

These proteins in gluten are what make pizza dough so pliable, and pastries so light and fluffy. You need gluten to keep dough together when you're trying to twist it into something delicious. Gluten is a binding agent that keeps your bread products together instead of having a crumbly mess. The proteins make your dough easy to work with and are essential in baked goods. These same proteins can be found in barley and rye and the unholy marriage of rye and wheat—triticale. It is believed a similar peptide chain can be found in oats, but it's not exactly the same thing. This is why some experts say celiacs cannot have oats, and others deem oats to be okay in small doses (as long as they are not processed with wheat flour). If you're suffering from symptoms of celiac disease, it would be best to put down the gluten-free oats until your gut is healed, just in case. No need to anger the villi.

Gluten is also a thickening agent, which is why you find "secret" gluten in marinades, flavored syrups, and salad dressings, even when there is no bread to be seen. Gravy, roux, and other sauces rely on gluten to provide that thick, smooth texture we all love. Even a thin-looking sauce could have a tiny amount of flour mixed in just to help the consistency. And just that tiny amount of flour will make the intolerant very, very sick.

This is why gluten is such a popular protein found in processed foods. Creating a pleasant texture, binding your protein bars together, and keeping food shelf stable are important when you're selling processed food. Gluten can help out in all of those areas. This is also why you have to read every single label of every single food found in a package, and sometimes you even have to call the manufacturer if you don't recognize an ingredient on the label of a food product. Gluten hides out, and you have to learn how to find it.

Some other ingredients containing gluten in processed foods include:

Barley
Rye
Triticale
Semolina
Bran
Spelt
Brewer's yeast
Hydrolyzed wheat protein
Malt (such as barley malt, malted milk, malted
    vinegar; anything unless it's specifically corn
    malt)
Oat flour
Matzo
Graham
Seitan
Bulgur
Farro

Beer

Farina

Einkorn

Bleached flour/unbleached flour

Filler (unless specified as corn)

Groats

Wheat germ

Soy sauce

Teriyaki sauce

Ponzu sauce

Orzo

Tabouli

Udon

It's the Processing and GMOs, Right?

As someone who prefers to have easily identifiable food, I can see how it would be easy to make genetically modified organisms the enemy. After all, those of us with food issues want to know exactly what's going into our bodies so we don't get sick. Unfortunately, this issue isn't relevant to this particular conversation, even though, yes, we would all do well to know exactly what we're eating at all times. If it were as easy as taking GMOs out of our diet, I would have been healed a few years ago, but alas, GMO-free gluten is still gluten.

There is also a lot of chatter about maybe just remov-ing that one protein, or perhaps that one protein doesn't exist in ancient grains, so let's eat that way and feel all right! Again, it would be great if we could solve the gluten problem so easily, but it's also not relevant. The fact is, if you have celiac disease, you have to avoid wheat/barley/rye, wheat/barley/rye products, and anything that touches wheat, barley, or rye. Yes, even organic, ancient wheat wearing a toga. It will mess you up, and big time. It's all about the gluten. Period.

For the Rest of the Gluten Avoiders

Now a word for our athletes who go gluten-free for performance reasons. There are a lot of you out there, and you seem to be winning tournaments, pennants, and accolades. Good job! I wish the rest of us gluten-free types could do the same. While simply going gluten-free won't transform an average athlete into a superstar, removing gluten from the athlete's diet is similar to adopting a high-protein/low-carb diet. Unless you keep eating all of those gluten-free packaged cookies. Before you go gluten-free, you should read on, as anyone adopting this diet should have an understanding of what gluten is and how it affects the body.

If you're getting your energy from the complex carbohydrates of vegetables instead of from breads, crackers, and pasta, you're getting fiber and nutrients that will help your body run properly and maintain your glucose levels in a healthy manner. If you're an athlete, you're certainly trying to make your body as healthy and strong as possible for peak performance. While some marathon runners eat a huge bowl of refined carbohydrates like pasta before a race, other athletes find that limiting their gluten (refined carbohydrates) helps their performance.

I have included some high-protein recipes because I know that a high-protein diet filled with vegetables so you still get energy from complex carbohydrates would actually get us all closer to looking like Venus Williams than we currently do. It is a healthy way to eat, it will give you loads of strength and endurance, and you will kick your sugar habit, which will go a long way in helping you win a race.

This is the reason I don't balk when people who don't have to go gluten-free do go gluten-free. Whether it's because you're going Paleo or living on a plant-based diet without gluten, it's a healthy choice. Unless you're just cutting out gluten and not eating a balanced diet, or replacing gluten-filled items with gluten-free items, such as brownies, pastas, and other carb- and sugar-loaded foods. Then your body is going to miss out on those vitamins it desperately needs, and you won't feel like a gluten-free superstar. You'll just be paying a lot more for groceries and wondering why you're gaining weight. If you're making a choice to go gluten-free as a diet or for health reasons, remember that other grains that replace gluten, such as rice flours, are not as good for your body as whole wheat. And if you don't really understand what gluten is, what it does, and how gluten does not simply = carbs, you're going to be disappointed with the results.

Before you dismiss those who go gluten-free for non-medical reasons, you should know that a lot of people say that a gluten-free diet does have the potential to give you more energy, make you more focused and physically stronger, and help your body function more efficiently. I say, more power to you, gluten-free enthusiasts. Welcome to the club.

Why All the Hate?

I'm not blaming the gluten-free by choice for 100 percent of this, but the fact is, there is a gluten-free backlash going on. This can make it difficult to explain to friends, family, and waiters why you're not eating the unlimited bread sticks anymore. You'll get a little bit of "That's horrible!!!" and a lot of the "So what CAN you eat?" business for a while. It's also possible you'll get a lot of incredulous looks, scoffs, and guffaws from people who just don't like what you're up to with this gluten shunning. The next time someone gives you the side eye when you tell them you have to eat gluten-free, just rattle off all the ailments gluten is responsible for in your particular body. I'm sure that unpleasant conversation will come to a quick halt.

Wait, Why Am I Giving Up Bagels Again?

Unless you've been hurling/vacating your bowels/sleeping for days/itching and require the gluten-free diet, you may be wondering if giving up your favorite foods is a good idea after all. I'm talking to you, the folks who are dipping your toe into the gluten-free experiment without a doctor's note. It's okay. Come on in.

Some of you have come to the gluten-free diet on your own or on the advice of a friend who has told you going gluten-free worked wonders for her body/mind/skin/social life. Others of you may have a family member who is gluten-free and you want to make it easier on that family member by going gluten-free yourself.

The short answer to "Why should I give up gluten if I'm not intolerant/allergic/celiac/immune-system compromised?" is that it's possible you shouldn't. There are nutrients in whole grains that help your body chug along, and if you remove those nutrients without keeping a sharp eye on your health, you could become deficient in certain vitamins and minerals. This is more likely to occur if you're not under a doctor's care with one of the issues that would cause you to benefit from a gluten-free diet. You need fiber as well, and if you're cutting out whole grains that contain gluten, you've got to replace fiber elsewhere. Unless you have an illness or a negative reaction to a food, you really shouldn't cut it out until you're fully educated and able to replace the nutrients you'll lose by cutting it out of your diet.

With that said, gluten is a difficult protein for everyone to digest. If you subscribe to the Paleo line of thinking, our bodies did not ingest gluten until the agriculture age, and therefore we are not evolutionarily equipped to handle it. I know that my husband, who has no gluten issues, has more difficulty digesting gluten now that we're a mostly gluten-free household. His body got "out of practice," and now he can feel it when he indulges in the occasional gluten-filled dinner outside our home. So yes, you may feel better by kicking gluten out of your diet. And if you do, I will not call you out as a fraud and an interloper, because I want as many gluten-free people out there requesting gluten-free options as possible. Also, who am I (who is anyone?) to say what you should and should not eat when you sit down in a restaurant and plan on paying good money for a meal? Who am I to judge what you serve at your dinner table?

When someone else makes a dietary choice, be it gluten-free, vegan, Paleo, sugar-free, alcohol-free, or whatever is floating that person's boat, it's not about me. It's not about you. It's about the person who is eating. And unless that person is causing a scene, judging you for not eating exactly like he is, or otherwise being a jerk about it, who cares? I certainly don't.

Trying out the gluten-free diet to see if you feel better is no different from trying out a Pilates class to see if your average-ish butt will turn into a rock-hard booty. We, especially Americans, are always in search of a better way to eat, exercise, be, and live. I don't know if it's our pioneer background, but we just can't seem to stop trying new things. Right now it's the gluten-free diet, and that's handy, since there are actually millions of undiagnosed celiacs running around out there. Perhaps some of you will come to the gluten-free diet because of the trend and discover that it's what you need in order to live a full and healthy life. Welcome, my rice-eating friends.

With that said, here is one piece of advice I hope everyone follows, gluten-free by choice or by prescription: Don't be a jerk about it. Don't cause a scene. Don't judge others. Oh, and if you are gluten-free by choice, don't get sloppy when you're dining out and make the chef and staff think that gluten-free is just a fad. That hurts the rest of us.

Myths and Truths About Gluten

Ever since gluten found its way into the national conversation, a heck of a lot of people have something to say about those proteins found in wheat, barley, rye, and triticale. Unfortunately, a lot of people don't actually know what they're talking about, or they heard it from a friend who . . . heard it from a friend who . . .

No worries, my friends! I'm here to set the record straight on all things gluten. Or most things gluten, I'm still not a scientist even though I've read enough medical terminology about gluten peptides to make me even more confused about whether I should be using the word "peptide," "protein," or "gliadin" or "glutenin." (Don't worry—I consult experts before I go on the Internet swearing that vodka is gluten-free.) So rather than listening to a Lohan or a McCarthy on the topic, allow me to drop some truth bombs on you about gluten.

MYTH: GOING GLUTEN-FREE MAKES YOU LOSE WEIGHT

You've heard this out of the mouths of many a celebrity who is asked to explain her sudden weight loss or stunning figure, so it totally must be true. If only you don't eat gluten, you, too, can look like Miley Cyrus! That is, if you want to.

TRUTH: GLUTEN-FREE SUBSTITUTIONS CAN MAKE YOU FAT

There are a number of celebrities out there making the "I got skinny going gluten-free" claim, which is how the message gets spread so far and wide. After all, a celiac named Mimi from Nebraska who gained weight after going gluten-free does not make it onto TMZ. But let's put this "gluten-free diet" trend into perspective. There's been this diet that rises and falls in popularity every other decade or so called the low-carb diet, or the South Beach Diet, or the Atkins Diet, depending on the era. It is a diet that cuts out carbs and sugars, and yes, you will lose weight if you go on this diet. And yes, gluten is found in foods that are carbohydrates. But that's where the connection ends.

If you go on a gluten-free diet for weight loss, you'll have to cut out gluten-free substitutes, too. That's because sugar is not good for a diet, so when you're subbing gluten-free brownies for gluten-filled brownies, you're not doing your waistline any favors. In fact, depending on the flour that is used in your gluten-free treats, you may be adding more sugar to your diet, not less. Rice flours, tapioca flours, and other gluten-free flours have more carbs and less nutritional value than whole wheat flours (although sorghum flour is a much better gluten-free choice), and you will not lose weight, and will probably even gain weight if you're substituting an all-purpose gluten-free flour in your recipes.

So don't listen to celebrities touting a diet du jour, and remember that they also have personal trainers and the means to overhaul their very famous bodies into any shape possible.

MYTH: YOU'RE LUCKY IF YOU HAVE CELIAC OR GLUTEN INTOLERANCE—IT'S SO TRENDY!

Wow, everywhere you go now has gluten-free options! And all you have to do is just not eat one thing in order to be healthy. You're soooooo lucky you got this disease/disorder.

TRUTH: CELIAC, ALLERGIES, AND GLUTEN SENSITIVITY ARE LIFELONG CONDITIONS THAT REQUIRE TREATMENT

While a part of me hopes the gluten-free diet isn't a short-lived trend, I know that, like most trendy diets, it will have its day and then everyone will forget about cutting out gluten except for those of us who still have to maintain this diet in order to be well. I don't know what the future holds for the gluten-free food market, but I do hope that with the increase in diagnoses, the demand will still be great enough to keep us in gluten-free options at the grocery store and when we dine out.

And yes, it *is* lucky that gluten-free is getting attention so that those of us who have to eat this way have more options. I feel for those who were diagnosed pre-2010, when few people knew what gluten was, and the gluten-free bread was inedible.

Of course, the gluten-free diet is only part of what we have to do to keep safe and healthy. For most of us, we're also battling vitamin and mineral deficiencies and other side effects—like bone density loss and anemia—as part of this disease. So while initially it is as "simple" as following the gluten-free diet, we also have to be mindful of our intake of other nutrients in order to keep our compromised bodies running smoothly so we don't fall prey to another illness.

MYTH: GOING GLUTEN-FREE WILL MAKE YOU A TENNIS STAR

Look at all of these Olympic medal winners with their gluten-free diets! And it's a fact that Novak Djokovic credits his gluten-free diet with helping him take home all those Grand Slams and Masters titles. If that's all it takes, I'm going to start training now and be ready to try out in two years.

TRUTH: YOU HAVE TO BE A TENNIS STAR FIRST BEFORE GOING GLUTEN-FREE

Adopting a gluten-free diet won't make you more athletic, attractive, run faster, or win gold medals. If you already have athletic talent, yes, you should follow a healthy, vitamin-packed diet for optimum performance. Again, a carb-free diet might help you feel healthier and keep in fighting form . . . maybe. But for us regular people, well, gluten-free isn't going to take us to the next level. Taking care of our bodies, getting plenty of exercise, and maybe taking a tennis class or two will be good for the gluten-free. But unless you started practicing when you were eight years old, don't count on any Wimbledon wins.

MYTH: GLUTEN INTOLERANCE IS ALL IN YOUR HEAD

You just know that if your friend could relax and stop stressing out about all of this stuff, her symptoms would simply go away. And you're sure that telling your friend to "just relax" is totally the answer. You're helping!

TRUTH: GLUTEN INTOLERANCE IS ALL IN YOUR GUT (AND OTHER PLACES)

Anyone who has experienced any of the symptoms of celiac or gluten intolerance knows it's not psychosomatic. Cramps, gastrointestinal distress, eczema, brain fog (okay, so that IS literally in your head), joint pain, and fatigue are real, physical symptoms that can happen when you ingest gluten. Historically, when doctors could not diagnosis a patient (especially a female patient), the answer was "stress" or "hysteria," if you want to go way back to Victorian times. And while having to race to a bathroom in the middle of a night out is certainly stressful, that urgency is not in your head but rather somewhere farther south. Also, when we are told that these painful, chronic physical symptoms are all in our heads, we want to do something to *your* head. And

it's not taking you out hat shopping. Please be respect-
ful to those of us in pain. After all, we only *wish* these
symptoms were in our head, so some therapy would
make them go away and we could eat normal pizza
again.

MYTH: A HUNDRED YEARS AGO, NO ONE WAS GLUTEN INTOLERANT

A century ago, everyone ate bread all the time and no
one was gluten intolerant. How is it possible that all of
these people are suddenly not able to eat something
that human beings have survived on for centuries with
no problem whatsoever?

TRUTH: YOUR GREAT-GRANDMOTHER WAS GLUTEN INTOLERANT

In my family, there is a history of gastrointestinal problems, some resulting in death, that went undiagnosed
for years. My own mother went undiagnosed with gluten ataxia and suffered dire consequences as a result of
going untreated for far too long. Autoimmune diseases
have consistently destroyed my family members' well-
being, yet I was the first person in my family to be
tested for celiac disease and put on a gluten-free diet.
The truth is, doctors know a lot more about celiac disease and gluten reactions today than they did 100, 50,
even 15 years ago. In fact, in North America, it was believed that celiac disease didn't even exist. This belief
has gradually changed over the past 20 years. That's
right, 20 years. The increase in diagnosis is because of
education and awareness, and it's all very, very recent.

There are still millions of people in North America who have not been diagnosed with celiac due to a lack of awareness. While this increase in celiac and gluten sensitivity diagnoses may not seem like a positive development, it is certainly a diagnosis many of our ancestors would have been more than happy to receive, and be treated for, without a doubt.

MYTH: IF A RESTAURANT HAS A GLUTEN-FREE MENU, YOU'RE SAFE

Huzzah! There's a gluten-free menu! You can sit back and relax and not worry about a thing.

TRUTH: YOU STILL HAVE TO HAVE THE CROSS-CONTAMINATION CONVERSATION

Thanks to the trendiness of the gluten-free diet, restaurants all over America are offering a gluten-free menu for those of us with issues. This is great news and will hopefully encourage celiacs, intolerants, and the allergic to dine out more often. Before you order from the gluten-free menu and consider yourself safe, however, take a minute to protect yourself. You still need to let your server know that you have a medical issue, and that is the reason you're ordering the gluten-free pizza crust. You need extra care with your order and need to make sure they aren't making your gluten-free version of dinner on the same counter as the gluten-filled version. That cross-contact with gluten will make you sick. (See Chapter 3, "Can't Someone Else Just Cook for Me?")

MYTH: EATING ANCIENT GRAINS AND BREADS FROM EUROPE WILL CURE CELIAC

You've heard the one about that one gluten intolerant who went to Europe and never had any problems eating that "pure European" bread? Oh, and Europeans just eat ancient grains and can digest breads with no problem. You should try it!

TRUTH: CELIACS CANNOT TOLERATE ANY WHEAT, REGARDLESS OF THE CENTURY OR COUNTRY OF ORIGIN

Wheat, no matter what kind, has those two proteins that cause the autoimmune response in those suffering from celiac disease. As long as gliadin and glutenin are present, celiacs are going to react negatively to ingesting wheat. It doesn't matter if it's an ancient grain or imported from the pristine bakeries of Switzerland, gluten is gluten is gluten. The high number of celiacs and gluten-intolerant Europeans should be proof enough that their bread, even if it is fresher and tastes a heck of a lot better than a loaf of all-American Wonder Bread, is still harmful.

MYTH: MONSANTO IS MAKING US ALL GLUTEN INTOLERANT

Genetically modified food is clearly the devil. If they would stop messing with food and making weird hybrids, using chemicals to make superfoods that yield high quantities, and generally being horrible bullies, these food intolerances would disappear.

TRUTH: GLUTEN INTOLERANCE WAS AROUND LONG BEFORE MONSANTO

There is an entirely separate debate to be had about our food being messed with in the form of genetically modified organisms and factory farming. Currently, Monsanto is the company many people identify as the evil empire that is modifying our food and contributing to an unhealthy population. Without stepping into this debate, I will say that we do know that whole, organic foods that are not altered in any genetic or chemical way are the best foods for our bodies. Gluten intolerance and celiac disease, however, were problems before our food chain became a science experiment, and we will continue to have the problem even if our food supply is clean.

MYTH: YOU CAN CHEAT ON YOUR GLUTEN-FREE DIET

What's the big deal with a cheat every now and then? At the least, we should be able to celebrate one "Waffle Wednesday" per month. Right?

TRUTH: THERE ARE NO "CHEAT" DAYS ON THE GLUTEN-FREE DIET

For any of us who have done the Whole30 or a grapefruit diet or two, you know that if you have a "cheat" day, nothing dramatic is going to happen other than feeling guilty and very disappointed in yourself. Not so with the gluten-free diet if you have an intolerance, an allergy, or celiac disease. Cheating and eating gluten means your body will be under attack. You will experience immediate physical symptoms, and you will be putting your health at risk. There are real consequences for ignoring the gluten-free diet that go far beyond one day.

MYTH: A LITTLE GLUTEN IS WORTH THE TUMMY ACHE

Why not taste that triple caramel cake that everyone is talking about? Just one bite won't hurt you, and you'll have the pleasure of feeling "normal."

TRUTH: EVEN A LITTLE GLUTEN CAUSES A BIG PROBLEM

Just like the cheat day, even a tiny bit of flour will damage your body. Sure, your symptom might be a tummy ache, but it's most likely much worse. You may also have debilitating joint pain, severe cramping, brain fog, and exhaustion—and you will most definitely put yourself at risk for malnutrition, cancer, and osteoporosis. As someone who has lost weeks because of an accidental ingestion of gluten and sits around worrying about developing a deadly disease, nothing is worth a little gluten. Nothing.

MYTH: IF YOU TELL A WAITER YOU'RE GLUTEN-FREE, HE'LL GIVE YOU EXTRA GLUTEN

Once you're gluten-free, you should never dine out. Waiters are incompetent at best and prone to mischief at worst. It's not worth the risk.

TRUTH: YOUR SERVER WANTS TO MAKE YOU HAPPY

Your waiter is there to help facilitate a happy dining experience for you. Happy dining experience = bigger tip. Additionally, people who work in the service industry have a much better night when their patrons are happy. I'm not sure when these rumors started about everyone in the service industry hating their jobs and their clientele, but it's pretty insulting to people who work in hospitality. And it's not true.

Sure, incompetent waiters do exist. But don't assume your waiter is going to harm you before you even walk into a restaurant. Be kind and polite, and you'll win over any waiter. Speak clearly, and explain what needs to happen in order for you to dine safely in the restaurant, then sit back and enjoy your evening out of the house. Trust in humanity. You'll be glad you did.

·TWO·

A Quick Lesson in What Foods to Avoid and What to Eat Instead

· · · · · · ·

Now that you know the dangers of gluten, it's time to create a safe space in your kitchen and in your car when you give in to the drive-thru on a Monday night when everything has gone wrong and, no, you are NOT going home to make a gourmet meal. We'll discuss dining out in the next chapter, but in the meantime, let's be crystal clear—*you can no longer allow McDonald's in your home.* I mean, you shouldn't for a lot of other reasons, but gluten is crawling all over that joint.

Of course, the Golden Arches' Happy Meal isn't the only food you'll have to ditch; there are many other delicious favorites that must be dismissed as well. Your home is the first line of defense of your belly, so let's start there. This is the area where you do have total control, and you should keep your kitchen 100 percent gluten-free. As someone who lives with three other people who *can* eat gluten, I know how challenging this can be. But we're talking about your health and well-being here, not about someone's preference for gluten-filled English muffins when there are perfectly good gluten-free versions available that will not make you sick for three days.

If you must allow any gluten into your home, treat it as the invader that it is: Quarantine that gluten. Have a designated pan for cooking any gluten, and never, ever use it to prepare your own foods. In fact, don't even allow it to be washed with the same scrub brush. Have a designated bowl, plate, cutting board, and toaster for the gluten as well. If you're sharing a toaster (which I don't recommend), wrap the gluten in foil before it goes in so that crumbs won't get everywhere, effectively contaminating your gluten-free goodies. Again, wash these items separately so the sticky gluten doesn't get all over your safe zones.

Everyone in your household must follow these safety rules if you're going to allow gluten inside your home. Gluten is a sneaky, sticky substance that can make many of us ill by ingesting the smallest amount. So quarantine your kitchen, or simply keep that gluten out.

Here are the sources of gluten you will have to clear out of your cupboards (the gluten-free versions are excepted, obviously):

Breads
Cereals
Pasta
Ramen
Bread crumbs
Pizza

Deep-fried anything in a batter

Pastries

Soy sauce

Barley malt (found in coffee syrups, sweeteners, salad dressing, and more)

Wheat vinegar (found in some of your favorite sushi restaurants)

Gravy

Oatmeal

Cake and cupcakes

Cookies

Crackers

Pies

Quiches

Hamburger and hot dog buns

Flour coating of anything

Candies thickened with flour

Pancakes and waffles

Graham crackers

Semolina

Bran

Einkorn

Kamut

Matzo

Processed meats

Beer

Malt liquor

Spelt

Chicken, beef, and vegetable broth (some brands)

Seitan

Couscous

Farro

Veggie burgers (some brands)

So that was a load of bad news. Let's move on to what you CAN eat without eating gluten, because it's pretty great. Naturally gluten-free foods include:

Dairy (cheese, milk, yogurt, butter, ice cream without add-ins)
Meats
Fish
Corn tortillas
Beans
Legumes
Eggs
Vegetables—all of them!
Fruits—all of them, too!
Corn
Quinoa
Buckwheat
Flax
Chia
Arrowroot
Gluten-free oats (in small amounts)
Millet
Sorghum
Soy (not soy sauce, just soy)
Amaranth
Teff
Nuts
Rice
Potatoes
Coffee
Wine
Spirits (vodka, bourbon, gin, tequila, etc.)

And don't forget about all of those gluten-free products now on the market, including pastas, desserts, and beer! (See Resources.) I don't know about you, but I could have a bang-up good time with all of those foods. I mean, not all at once, but there's enough deliciousness to go around without gluten. Just flip over to the 30-day meal plan and my 100 recipes and you'll see how easy it can be to live the G-free life.

Yes, I know that some of you are also ditching the dairy and other foods as well. While that's certainly more challenging, it is not impossible. You've just got to get creative with your menu. And remember, your food choices should be based on health—not trends. If you feel worse while following a specific diet, talk to your doctor and find out what is best for your body.

A Word About Grain-Free

There are those who say a grain-free diet is the way to go for optimum health, especially if you have a gluten problem. The Paleo diet, specifically, is an incredibly popular way to eat for people who are also avoiding gluten and love their (grass-fed, organic, antibiotic-free) meat. What this means is that you're giving up gluten (wheat, barley, rye, triticale) as well as all the other grains out there (rice, corn, buckwheat, quinoa, millet, sorghum, tapioca, etc.). While I'm a fan of not cutting out even one more thing in my diet, I do go grain-free on occasion just for the heck of it. I mean, it's not going to kill me, and it usually means fewer calories. I also notice that if I restrict my diet after accidental gluten ingestion, I tend to heal faster. This is *my* experience, not a scientific fact, so again, listen to your own body and follow your doctor's advice when eating for health. Given the popularity of this movement, and my own occasional dipping into the Paleo, I have provided some grain-free recipes for those who are leaning that way.

Wait, So What's Paleo? And Why Should I Care?

Paleo eating has gotten super popular, and I can see why. Not only is this diet loosely based on what our ancestors ate (grass-fed organic meat, no grains, no dairy, no refined sugar, lots of vegetables, minimal fruit, absolutely nothing processed), but also everyone and her sister has lost weight while chowing down on steak. I get it. In fact, I do go Paleo every now and then and sometimes even take it into Whole30 territory. (The Whole30 way of eating is 30 days of extreme Paleo— in addition to living *la vida Paleo*, remove any natural sugars, booze, all legumes, potatoes, soy, and fruit juice, and eat only whole foods.) When you have an autoimmune disease like celiac, going on an anti-inflammatory diet like the Whole30/Paleo can be good for your system. It's not sustainable—for me, anyway, because I know I'm weak and I love cheese—but it can be like pushing a reset button.

There are people who say eating that much meat (with fat included) cannot possibly be good for your heart and cholesterol. While the latest studies have shown the "fat" argument to be flawed, again, don't start a diet without consulting your doctor.* What works for the Paleo crowd may not work for you. I will

---

* "Ending the War on Fat," *Time*, June 12, 2014, time.com/2863227/ending-the-war-on-fat.

say I feel better when removing certain foods from my diet, but I've never done Paleo or the Whole30 long term, so my experience is just that—only mine.

Gluten-Free Pasta and You

Even those who are not forced to go gluten-free can't help noticing the expansion of the gluten-free pasta section in the grocery store. What began as a little pile of brown rice pasta has grown to include gluten-free grains such as quinoa, corn, and millet, as well as lentils and black beans. You can buy everything from macaroni to lasagna, fresh or dried. It's a crowded pasta field out there, and as such, it can be incredibly confusing.

What's also confusing is the proper way to cook gluten-free pasta. Unlike the white flour pastas, gluten-free versions present a host of challenges. You don't want to cook your gluten-free brown rice pasta for too long or it will turn into mush. If you don't cook your gluten-free quinoa pasta long enough, it will break your teeth. Before you bust out your favorite carbonara recipe, follow this gluten-free pasta advice:

1. **Follow the package directions to the letter.** That is, unless you've found your favorite pasta and it tastes right only if you cook it for 5 minutes instead of 7. Some like al dente, and some like a little give. But in order to avoid a giant pile of mush, never overcook your pasta, and stir it a few times while it's cooking to keep it separated.

2. **Experiment with gluten-free grains.** In the beginning of my gluten-free cooking journey, I hated corn

pasta and swore by brown rice pasta. Now you can't get me away from the corn pasta and even the quinoa (which I also swore off after a particularly bad batch). If you're making a pasta salad, try the lentil or black bean versions for something completely different. Your tastes will change, so always be ready to try something new.

3. **Change your pasta with each recipe.** While I love an al dente corn macaroni when I make a casserole, I prefer a brown rice spaghetti when I'm using only a few ingredients. You don't have to always go with one grain, so mix it up!

4. **Don't be afraid of the water.** A lot of gluten-free pastas begin "shedding" as they cook. What you get next is a load of cloudy water, which can look frightening and a bit strange. Don't worry! It's totally normal.

Dairy: The Oft-Maligned Nectar of the Gods

So many of you know that those of us with gluten problems can often develop dairy problems as well. While I've never met a milkshake that is my friend, as long as I'm not doing that Paleo thing, I still do eat cheese, butter, and other dairy products that aren't straight-up milk to my gut. I have, however, experimented with alternative milks and nondairy options in my cooking since I know so many of you have this issue. Many of my recipes are dairy-free or can easily be made dairy-free. Substitute almond milk in almost any recipe and it will work just fine. Experiment with ghee instead of butter, and feel free to skip the cheese. Nutritional yeast is a great substitute for Parmesan if you're adding flavor to your roasted vegetables or want to dress up your kale chips or popcorn. And I'm saying this as a die-hard cheese lover. While I will love dairy until I die, I realize it does not love a lot of us back.

I've also noticed that if I've accidentally ingested gluten, dairy makes my recovery time last longer and makes me much more uncomfortable. So I feel your dairy-free pain (sometimes) and want to help you through it. No matter how much I want to drive-thru and get a black-and-white shake at In-N-Out.

Which Brings Us to the Vegan Conversation

I know, love, and respect many a vegan and have tried it out myself a few times. When I cut out the animal products, I lose weight, my skin clears up, and my stomach is pretty darn happy. My head and heart, however, get kind of angry. I believe you should consider food not only as a way to fuel your body (and in the case of us gluten haters, to heal the body), but also as something to truly enjoy. I have had *many* vegan dishes that I not only enjoy but also re-create in my kitchen as often as possible. Additionally, when I'm on a vegan kick, I feel like I can look at my dog without guilt, knowing I'm on her team. Still, there's something missing for me when I follow a plant-based diet. I'm not saying that going vegan is necessarily an act of deprivation, but I do often feel deprived when I eat this way. Which, when you're already on a medically restricted diet, does not feel great. So I go "occasional vegan" and try to be mindful about what I'm putting into my body, with the main exception being Deep-Fried Chocolate Cream Cookies (see the recipe on page 210).

Whole Foods vs. Cheetos

While a lot of people ditch gluten and try to live on a whole-food-only diet, the fact is that sometimes processed gluten-free treats are a delicious way to feel normal for a quick minute. I find that I get frustrated trying to read too many packages wrapped around my gluten-free foodstuffs and tend to head toward the outer aisles of my local grocery stores as often as possible. And while some companies *are* labeling whole foods with a "gluten-free" stamp (Ummm, butter? Seriously?), it's much easier to grab a head of broccoli and a grass-fed steak and know that you'll be able to have a safe dinner. It's also better for the sensitive to eat whole foods rather than a combination of who knows what. So make it your goal to eat mostly whole foods and relegate anything in a package to a sometimes food.

Of course, "sometimes" happens more often when you're eating on the go, on vacation, or just crunched for time. Because it happens to all of us, we need to learn how to read the labels on packaged foods so we can eat safely.

The Food Allergen Labeling and Consumer Protection Act (FALCPA) was passed by the U.S. Congress in 2004, but it has taken until recently (2013, to be exact, with a full year given to companies to comply) to fully implement. Today in the United States, food must be labeled if it contains one of the top eight allergens (milk, soy, wheat, peanuts, tree nuts, eggs, fish, and shellfish). The definition of gluten-free food under this act is food that contains less than 20 parts per million of gluten, which has been the standard measure for tolerance among the celiac population. While this certainly should make all of us feel much better, keep in mind that unless a packaged food has been certified gluten-free, it can be manufactured in a facility that also processes gluten-containing foods, thereby increasing the potential for cross-contact with gluten. I know it's frustrating, but we've made a lot of progress in just the last decade.

Luckily, the market for gluten-free food is expanding by the second, and you can find just about anything to substitute for your gluten-filled favorites that is fully gluten-free, made in a gluten-free facility, and safe for celiac sufferers. And if you can't, check out Chapter 8, where I teach you how to make your own chicken Parmesan and grilled cheese delights. You'll be satisfied in no time.

In the meantime, here's a handy list to show you what to grab when all you want is gluten. (See Chapter 8 and Resources for these fantastic swaps.)

REPLACE THIS WITH THAT

- Donuts = Glutino Gluten-Free Toaster Pastry
- Burger and fries = Ever had a GF Truffle Cheeseburger? You won't go back to gluten.
- Cheerios = Yes, they do make Gluten-Free Whole O's!
- Cookies 'n' cream ice cream = Ice Cream Pecan Ball or So Delicious GF/DF cookies 'n' cream ice cream
- Chicago deep-dish pizza = Lou Malnati's Gluten-Free Thin Crust Pizza
- Croissant = Gluten-free beignets
- Fried calamari = Did you know that cornstarch is better for deep-frying? You do now.
- Kit Kat/Twix/your favorite candy bar = Andy's Dandy Candy Bars

- Sweet and sour chicken = Wouldn't you rather have *The Gluten-Free Cheat Sheet* recipes and actually know what's in your favorite dish?
- Fried chicken and waffles = Fry up your own gluten-free chicken and add my GF Ham and Cheese Waffles for double the pleasure.
- Deep-fried Oreos = Gluten-free deep-fried chocolate cream cookies. You guys, there are now *four* kinds of gluten-free Oreo-like cookies! Let's fry 'em.

Grocery Stores for the Gluten-Free

Only a few years ago, if you wanted gluten-free foods, you had to find a specialty store or spend your entire paycheck at Whole Foods. While I still love to hang out at Whole Foods (their gluten-free in-house par-baked bread products are fantastic), the reality is that every single grocery store you walk into today will carry some gluten-free items. If not an entire gluten-free section, you'll be able to find gluten-free crackers and cookies tucked into the aisles with the regular products. And of course, naturally gluten-free foods have been there all along. Check out Resources for my favorite gluten-free products to help get your shopping started.

Gimme Drugs

One area that could trip up even the most vigilant gluten-free gal is the one that isn't even something you eat. I'm talking about vitamins and prescription and over-the-counter medications. It's true, some meds and vitamins contain gluten in the form of fillers and starch, and so you can't swallow a pill without knowing what's inside.

Additionally, those of us who have celiac disease must be vigilant about taking vitamins since we're most likely deficient in some areas. But you don't want to take vitamins to be healthy and end up glutening yourself. And since vitamins are something you should take every day, it's important that you know exactly what you're taking; otherwise, you won't heal up and will wonder why you keep getting sick even if you think you're following a gluten-free diet. This is, in fact, fairly common. Don't let it happen to you. I'm a big fan of Country Life vitamins since they're gluten-free, but there are other options as well. (See Resources.)

Prescription drugs can be very difficult to understand, so be sure you have the conversation with your prescribing doctor, your pharmacist, and even the manufacturer if you don't feel you have the right answers. You can also visit the website Glutenfreedrugs.com to check out prescription and over-the-counter medications, but first have a conversation with everyone who is dispensing the medication.

The same goes for over-the-counter medications. Check the label, talk to the manufacturer, go online if it's still not clear, *and* talk to a pharmacist. Take it from the lady who continually gluten-ed herself on a generic form of Tylenol—not all generics are created equal.

It Gets Better

If you're like me, you will spend the first few years of your gluten-free life living by that substitutes list. It's hard to give up your favorite foods, especially when it seems like everyone around you is Tweeting nonstop about the latest artisanal donut shop. Once you've indulged yourself to the point of saturation, it's time to head down a different aisle in the grocery store—the spice and gourmet sections.

Cooking with exciting and bold flavors is incredibly satisfying—more so than a quick fix of bread. Becoming a "fancy" cook by using only the finest ingredients will not only satisfy your need for delicious food, but make everyone around you clamor for your recipes. So plow through the spices, hit up your local ethnic food shops, grab some gourmet staples, and start experimenting with flavor. A little flavor goes a long way toward making you feel happy and full. Splurge on these fancy-pants foods to cook with and forget all about gluten:

Truffle salt
Saffron
Risotto
Spices to make curry/curry premade
Heirloom tomatoes
Kale, Swiss chard, and collard greens
Mesquite flour
Vietnamese cinnamon
Bourbon vanilla
Coconut cream
Farm-fresh, organic, free-range eggs (the fresher the better)
Duck eggs
Sriracha
Vanilla almond milk
High-quality dark chocolate
Grass-fed beef—any cut

Pasta Pairs

· · · · ·

Combine the following ingredients and gluten-free pastas for optimum pasta enjoyment:

Fresh corn fettuccine + butter, Parmesan,
salt, pepper, and broccoli

Brown rice spaghetti + chicken piccata

Quinoa macaroni + American cheese, cheddar
cheese, Parmesan, milk, and butter

Black bean pasta + salsa,
cheddar cheese, and avocado

Corn lasagna + marinara sauce, prosciutto,
ricotta cheese, and mozzarella

THREE

Can't Someone Else Just Cook for Me?

● ● ● ● ● ● ● ●

It's hard to know which bit of news is harder to hear when a doctor/friend/nutritionist/coach tells you to give up the gluten—that you can't eat bread sticks anymore or that you have to learn how to cook. I thank my grandmothers every day that I have a cooking gene somewhere deep down inside; otherwise, I might be living on gluten-free crackers with (wine and) cheese right now. Okay, so sometimes that *is* what I have for dinner, but being able to cook up a quick-and-easy gluten-free chicken piccata has saved many a day. And it will go a long way in your new gluten-free life as well.

I can hear those of you who use your kitchen as storage hissing at me as I type. Still, learning some basics about cooking will be absolutely necessary as you go gluten-free. I mean, unless you have a personal chef who also knows the difference between wheat and buckwheat (which is gluten-free!). But if you're like the rest of us, you're going to have to do your own gluten-free cooking at home, so the sooner you make peace with it, the better.

Did you catch that loophole? *At home . . .*

I'm about to make all of you in the Microwave Dinner Club very happy with this tip: In order to get someone else to make a delicious gluten-free dinner, you should just *leave the house.*

No, really, it's okay out there. Everyone and her Kardashian are avoiding gluten, so most restaurants will totally know what you're talking about. Sure, some will not, and we'll get to that later. But right now, let's talk about getting you out of the kitchen and allowing others to serve you. Yes you can!

Now that you've mastered the list of foods without gluten, start looking for restaurants that specialize in those foods, and start crossing off restaurants that have the letters *K, F,* and *C* in their name. There are certain types of food that are much more likely to be gluten-free friendly than others, so let's start at those delicious places, shall we? Keep your hungry eye out for the following cuisines:

Mexican. Traditional Mexican food uses a lot of corn, beans, meats, and vegetables. These are all your friends. Just beware of anything fried or rolled in a flour tortilla. I'm sorry to report that this includes tortilla chips. While most of your favorite Mexican restaurants will have a dedicated basket for cooking up these delicious crispy wonders, always ask if there is double dipping with flour tortillas going on in the fryer. A good way to know if the Mexican food joint is not you-friendly is to check and see if there is a "Tex" in front of the "Mex."

Those Tex-Mex guys love batter-dipped, flour-tortilla-wrapped dishes. Your gluten-free digestive system does not.

French. As long as you skip the baguette and sauces, French food is a good bet. Most classically trained chefs working in the French style keep ingredients simple, so you're less likely to get a mystery dish on your plate. If you also keep your order simple, you'll be in for a treat. That is, if your version of treat includes meat, cheese, vegetables, butter, and chocolate. Yum.

Vegetarian/Vegan. These are the people who watch what is in their food even more closely than we do. Dine out with the vegetarian and vegan populations, and you'll never have to guess what ingredients are on the menu. Of course, you've got to dodge any meat substitutes (seitan is not your friend) and whole grains that contain gluten, but most restaurants that pride themselves on being creative and healthy will have plenty of gluten-free options as well.

Sushi. With one *huge* caveat, sushi and sashimi are fantastic dinner options. Just call ahead to make sure they have wheat-free tamari available to substitute for soy sauce and that they don't douse everything with soy sauce before they even bring it out to your table. One more issue—some random sushi joints use wheat vinegar to cook the rice. Call the restaurant first and ask if they use wheat vinegar. If you're clear on both the soy sauce and the wheat vinegar fronts, go crazy! Some sushi restaurants even offer a rice flour tempura so you can revisit that old fried favorite.

American. What do Americans love? Meat and potatoes. As long as it's not all deep-fried (and this is not a given), burger joints and the like can be a safe haven for the gluten-free. Be careful at the burger joints, though, as cross-contamination could be a big problem if everything is getting cooked on the same surface. And always, always, always ask if the French fries have been dredged in flour or fried in the same basket with the onion rings, fish sandwiches, or anything else that uses flour. And here's another tip—many restaurants use frozen French fries from another source, so they have no idea what's in the mix. I would avoid those French fries, but if your heart is set on having those crispy 'taters, ask to see the bag they arrived in and check for any suspicious ingredients. Oh, and the condiments on the table? You're safe using everything that does not include "malt" ingredients. Yes, even the mustard, as long as it's not fancy "house-made" mustard that uses beer as an ingredient.

Ethiopian. A giant piece of gluten-free *injera* bread topped with lentils, meats, greens, and other legumes is a typical meal at an Ethiopian restaurant. All of which is safe for the gluten-free diner. Just beware, as some restaurants may add white flour in with the traditional teff used to make injera. Always ask before you dig in.

Seafood. Unless you're going to a fish fry, checking into a fresh seafood restaurant is an excellent choice for the gluten-free. Seafood tastes best when it's prepared with very few ingredients, and great chefs will not mess with a great thing. Always beware of the bread crumbs, and go forth and cast your line.

Italian. Aha! Gotcha there, didn't I? I used to write off Italian restaurants because not being able to eat ravioli made me sad. Not unlike the population of Italy itself, many Italian restaurants are getting with the gluten-free program and, in addition to having meat and risotto dishes, are offering gluten-free pasta and pizza crusts. This is very exciting. And as long as you go through the cross-contamination drill (see page 47), you should be able to enjoy some red sauce outside of your home once again.

Of course, the great thing about this restaurant revolution we're happily in the middle of is that any type of food can be made gluten-free and a heck of a lot of restaurateurs are going there. Before you head out, check your local gluten-free blogger recommendations (see Resources) or simply Google "Gluten-free [name of your town]" and see what magic can happen. Remember, even with a glowing recommendation, a restaurant can change menus, managers, chefs, and attitudes at any time. It's always a good idea to call ahead and ask if there will be safe gluten-free options before you make a reservation or head across town.

Check Out Our New Gluten-Free Menu!

It seems like every time I step inside a chain restaurant in America, I find a gluten-free menu. This is awesome. This can also cause me to head to a known chain (see Resources) instead of taking a chance with a new farm-to-table joint. Sometimes. Having been served gluten at a restaurant with a clearly marked gluten-free menu, let me tell you that just because it's on a GF menu does not guarantee it's safe. You still have to go through the drill of asking the right questions, explaining your situation, and being vigilant even if there is a clearly marked menu.

I have one more piece of good news for you gluten-free types. As I write this, there are nine (9!) ShopHouse Southeast Asian Kitchen restaurants in the United States, with one more opening soon. Why is this Southeast Asian restaurant chain from the team behind Chipotle so exciting? It's not only 100 percent gluten-free, but also 100 percent dairy-free. Win. And win. While these restaurants are only in California and the Washington, DC, area right now, if we all go there, like, all the time, they will surely expand, so we can all know we have a safe and delicious option for lunch and dinner.

Meet Your New BFF—Your Waiter

Here's a truth I cannot repeat enough: Your waiter is the key to your good time. The person you talk to first, last, and throughout your meal is the person who keeps your dinner safe. A waiter who understands gluten and the seriousness of your situation is a waiter who deserves a big tip after you dine safely. You may have a chef who knows what she's doing in the kitchen but a waiter who doesn't understand what the heck he's doing up front. That's a recipe for disaster. On the flip side, I've had many a waiter save my entire night by being my advocate in the kitchen. You must communicate your needs thoroughly to the waiter and make sure he understands what you're saying.

One way you can know if your waiter "gets it" is if

he talks about how they don't use soy sauce in their dressings. That's a clued-in waiter. A waiter who isn't quite up to speed will probably think you can't have butter on anything and will deny you potatoes. *You have to educate your waiter in order to eat safely.* Consider it a favor to the next gluten-free diner sitting down at his station. After all, someone probably did it for you already.

By now your dining-out dance card might be pretty full. Before you go for it and start dialing up every place in town, we're going to have to have the cross-contamination conversation . . .

How to Ruin a Gluten-Free Meal

When I first heard about cross-contamination (some people more accurately call this cross-contact, by the way) while dining out, I decided it was only for neurotic people. I didn't care if a little gluten got close to my burger because I was not going to be one of those uptight gluten-free nags. I was going to be this new version of the cool gluten-free (note: This does not actually exist) and just roll with whatevs, man. Do you know how many times I got sick? *Every time.* Do you know how my villi looked when I went for my follow-up endoscopy? Shredded. I really don't want to get cancer, and I don't want you to get cancer either, so let's all work harder on making sure our food is safe.

It's a huge drag to have to make sure that a restaurant not only has gluten-free options on the menu, but also knows how to prepare that food safely. I mean, that's like five extra questions for that waiter! I hate this, and you'll probably hate it, too, but it's necessary for celiacs. (Gluten intolerants have a little more wiggle room here, but you should talk to your doctor and/or nutritionist before ditching the cross-contamination conversation.) But think of it this way: It's like avoiding "just a little" arsenic over a period of time. You may feel a tiny bit bad (or if you're like me, a horrible amount bad) by ignoring the situation, but over time you're going to lose your marbles—and a whole lot more. So have the conversation. Your gut/skin/joints/brain will thank you.

Here's what you have to consider when dining out, even if you're ordering gluten-free food:

- Is this corn tortilla being heated up on the same press as a flour tortilla?
- Is the gluten-free pasta being cooked in the same pot as the regular pasta?
- Was my burger cooked on the same grill as those toasted-up gluten-filled buns?
- Is my gluten-free pizza crust being cooked on the same surface as those gluten-y ones?
- Are you handling bread, then handling my gluten-free dinner?
- Did you just take the sandwich meat off that sour-dough roll and throw it on a plate?
- Is that a pita chip sticking out of my gluten-free hummus?

I'm sorry, but these are issues to be explored and questions that need to be asked when you dine out. I know. I wish we didn't have to either, but spending a birthday in bed and a Mother's Day in the bathroom taught me that you really can't cut corners here.

These Are the Food Culprits

Let's review the sneaky foods restaurants just might be adding to your gluten-free dinner without realizing it's going to bend you over faster than a Texas twister. Sadly, there are a lot of nasty, gluten-y additives and tricky ninja foods out there that chefs may use to flavor, thicken, or crisp up your restaurant meal. While you have already kicked these out of your home, they may not be obvious to anyone else preparing your dinner. These aren't the main ingredients in your dish; rather, they are items a chef may toss in as a helper. That's why you have to ask, since they're not likely to be listed on the menu. Watch out for:

Soy sauce
Barley malt
Malt vinegar
Wheat vinegar
A dusting of flour
Flour used on a surface for nonstick purposes
Malt in ice cream dishes
Bread crumbs (also panko—that's bread, too)
Beer
Mustard or marinades made with beer
Pita (I wouldn't be bringing this up if it hadn't
    happened to me. Yes, someone in the food
    service industry thought pita was not really
    bread and was therefore gluten-free.)

So now that you know what to look out for, prepare a speech. Just say this to your waiter: "Does this have any soy sauce, a dusting of flour, malt vinegar, malt balls, cookie dust; and did you fry it/cook it/boil it/grill it on the same surface/basket/pot/stone as something with gluten?"

Easy, right?

Now for the Bad News

Sometimes restaurants are simply not going to be safe for you. While we can hope these restaurants will be easily identifiable as such, and therefore you never step foot inside those deep-fried walls, that won't always be the case. Whether it's a friend's birthday or a family vacation, you will wind up in an unsafe environment at some point. There is not a heck of a lot you can do under these circumstances other than going into the bathroom and crying. Once you've dried your tears and have resigned yourself to starving for the evening, here's how to spend the other 1.5 hours at B.J.'s BBQ Emporium:

- Drink wine. (Note: Designated driver required, maybe even designated conversation monitor.)
- Grab that pack of gluten-free snacks you always carry on your person. (You do that, right?)
- Sneak out the back door and search the neighborhood for food and/or entertainment. Just make sure you're back in time for the singing of "Happy Birthday," "For He's a Jolly Good Fellow," and the like. (Note: This only works if you are not supposed to be the center of attention.)
- Comfort yourself knowing that you'll be stopping off for whatever the heck you want after enduring this entire meal while starving.

But seriously, if you do find yourself in a restaurant that doesn't listen to your needs, messes up an order after you repeatedly explain your situation, or is openly hostile—just leave. Your dinner companions should understand that your health is more important than decorum. And if they don't, well, maybe don't dine out with that crowd anymore.

You can dine out (mostly) safely, but you have to do your research and be willing to leave if you find yourself in a dangerous situation. It is mortifying to walk out of a restaurant (or it is for me, anyway), so that's why I'll at least look at a menu if I don't have a chance to call and talk gluten with the management. Minimizing your chances for failure is a very important task when you start to venture outside your home. It's true those spontaneous days of "Let's just see where we wind up for lunch!" are over. But those days of "Let's see how horrible I feel after dinner" will be over, too.

Even though we have to be incredibly cautious and advocate for ourselves constantly, it is getting so much easier to leave your home and get a good gluten-free meal. I probably dine out three or four times a week, and 99 percent of the time, it is 100 percent safe. That other 1 percent of the time? I have to crawl into bed for a week or two. I consider myself lucky to run into problems only sporadically and consider it the cost of not living my life under house (kitchen) arrest. If you're going for 100 percent, my friends, you will have to stay in your own safe kitchen. I would suggest, however, that you live a little. Just be smart, be prepared, and know when to get the heck out of Dodge.

FOUR

Depression, Anxiety, and General Crankiness

· · · · · · · ·

All this gluten talk is probably making you pretty cranky. I know it's making me cranky, and I'm a seasoned expert. Whether you're just upset about this big upheaval or you're in a much darker place, let's talk about it! There are two ways to look at depression, anxiety, and celiac. The clinical manner, and the "I'm so freaking tired of being sick!!!!" manner. Both are, of course, valid.

I know I get anxious every time I have to go to dinner at the home of someone I don't know very well. I tend to freak a little bit every time there's a school event that includes dinner right after work and I haven't had time to eat. And sure, every time we head to the airport or out of town, or out to dinner with new people or to a new restaurant, yep, I tense up and want to cry just a little. Okay, sometimes a lot. You can't get around the fact that celiac disease is incredibly anxiety-inducing.

I'm guessing that those of you who have a wheat allergy can knock that anxiety up a notch or five on account of the possible hospitalization and/or death angle, and those of you who are gluten intolerant have another level of anxiety, which is the "No one believes me, anyway . . ." kind of thing. Big sigh.

For me, and probably for many of you, the worst of the depression (clinical or not) and anxiety comes when somehow, some way, gluten has gotten into my body. This can take me to a dark place. First, I look at my calendar and work out what events/work/fun stuff/travel I can afford to cancel and what I have to make work, no matter how much I need to stay in the bathroom and then crawl under the covers. Depending on what that looks like (and let's face it, being a nonmillionaire without a household staff, I have a calendar that *never* looks manageable), I get seriously anxious or resign myself to a monthlong depression.

Next, while the symptoms are flowing through my body and making me miserable, I start to lose hope. I tend to forget that my stomach will stop screaming at me, my time spent in gastrointestinal distress will dramatically decrease, and at some point, I won't need to sleep for 10 to 12 hours every day. When you're in the middle of it, it's easy to lose hope and to focus on what else you're losing in the process (time, money, sanity). But things really get kicked into high gear when I start thinking about the side effects. And if my symptoms go on longer than usual, I can work myself up into an "I know this time it's cancer" situation. Yep, I go there.

What I'm trying to say here is that dealing with a chronic illness can make even the most positive person go to a deep, dark place and wallow around for a bit. I have, and I probably will again, even if I read this chapter over and over.

There is also a clinical angle to all these yucky feelings for some people with celiac disease. The autoimmune response caused by gluten is not limited to the gut. In addition to those people diagnosed with gluten ataxia (an autoimmune response that attacks the brain), celiacs can also have neurological symptoms. While my joints are being affected by inflammation due to my celiac disease, your brain might be experiencing a drop in endorphins and depression could set in. The good news is that, like with celiac disease, the cure is a gluten-free diet. And we all know what the bad news is: the gluten-free diet and those times that gluten slips in without us knowing.

As with all other illnesses, if your depression and anxiety are not improved by your gluten-free diet, don't assume it's part of the package. Talk to your doctor about getting help whether through medication, therapy, or a combination of both. It's true, those of us dealing with celiac disease do have a lot to get down about, but if depression has become your dominant state of being, please do seek help outside of just sticking to the gluten-free diet. Even if you don't think you fit the bill for clinical depression, it's always good to find support outside your own family to deal with challenging issues.

Will I Ever Feel Healthy Again?

This is the big one. When you are sick and suffering, it's hard to know there's an end in sight. Hope is hard to come by, and who has the energy for being all sunny and bright anyway? Because gluten happens. No matter how safe you are, somehow, someday, you will accidentally ingest gluten in spite of your best efforts. And if you're like me, just the tiniest speck can knock you down for weeks. Sometimes those weeks happen during a stressful time at work; sometimes they happen during the holidays when you're trying really hard to enjoy yourself. That's upsetting and, at the risk of sounding like my five-year-old, really unfair.

But now that you know how to minimize the possibilities of getting sick thanks to that villainous gluten, you will be feeling better, and you will begin to feel hope once again. If you aren't feeling better after kicking gluten out of your diet, you should talk with both your doctor and a nutritionist to see if something else is bothering your body and if you're taking in all the nutrients your body needs to stay healthy. While some people give up gluten and bounce back to health quickly, everyone is different and heals at different rates. Be patient with your body and take good care of yourself on this road to wellness.

If/when you do accidentally ingest gluten and find yourself sick again, know that you will come out of it again. Don't let one slipup become an excuse to binge on more gluten-filled foods. As I've learned the hard way, you're not going to get any better by treating your body even worse when it's in a weakened state. And even though it's crazy tempting to throw bad stuff down my gullet to help stuff the feelings of frustration, time has taught me to treat myself better than that.

When I get sick now, I may still mope around a bit, but honestly, it's like second nature at this point. I make sure to load up on probiotics and be more vigilant about taking my vitamins and eating right. Some people take activated charcoal pills (you can find these at health food stores) to help even out the gastrointestinal symptoms, and I try that sometimes as well if things are not moving along as quickly as I'd like. Drink plenty of water, get tons of rest, and it will pass. Don't worry, you'll be back out there rocking the GF lifestyle in no time. Or maybe in just a little time.

You've Gotta Have GFFs

Given all these challenges, it's a great idea to have a community around you to help you stay gluten-free. The sad fact is, no one who isn't experiencing your health issues is going to truly "get it" no matter how much he loves you. Even the best friend or significant other in the world might throw her hands up in the air the fiftieth time you need to vent about donuts. Again, I learned this the hard way.

Whether you're someone who likes a face-to-face meet-up or online chatting is more your thing, there are many organizations out there that support celiacs, and even more bloggers out there who will help you when you need a morale boost. There are conferences and gluten-free expos all over North America (and beyond if you're a world traveler) where you can meet other gluten-free people and sample the latest in gluten-free cuisine. (See Resources.) We are out there, and we are very welcoming. Join a group, read a blog, take a gluten-free vacation, and find friends who really get what it means to soldier through another gluten-filled wedding reception. You will find your gluten-free tribe, and you will start to feel like yourself again.

Leavening Things Up with a Bit of Humor

· · · · ·

Humor is subjective, but we all know when someone is being mean-spirited instead of hilarious. Just in case you're having trouble sorting out whether someone is laughing with you or at you, here are a few gluten humor dos and don'ts:

DO: Come up with a cute nickname for your gluten-free friend. While I certainly never mind being referred to as someone's "GFF" (gluten-free friend), I bet you can get even more creative and adorable. Like maybe "Queen-oa."

DON'T: Call someone a "glutard." I know some people with a terrific sense of humor who are gluten-free and call *themselves* "glutards." But don't assume we all appreciate a slang name that also plays off another population that certainly doesn't deserve to be insulted.

DO: Forward gluten-free memes and the like. I don't know how many people sent me the *Onion* article "How to Live Gluten-Free" (theonion.com/articles/how-to-live-glutenfree), and I shared it with even more of the gluten-free because it's hilarious. BuzzFeed has had some pretty great memes on what it's like to have to be gluten-free, and some gluten-free bloggers are great at rolling in the hilarious gluten-free gifs. These make us feel like we're all on the same team, and even if it's a sad team, we can laugh together because *we get it*.

DON'T: Forward insulting segments from late-night talk shows. Without trying to do that thing that is explaining why something is funny vs. being not-at-all funny, try to put yourself in our gluten-free shoes when you hear something on TV or the Internet. If the joke lies in making fun of the person who is gluten-free, that's not going to be funny to those of us who are the butt of the joke. Honestly, for all you comedians, would-be comedians, bloggers, talk show hosts, relatives, friends, coworkers, and anyone else who is considering making a funny joke about gluten, there are just two dos and don'ts when it comes right down to it:

DO: Be funny.

DON'T: Be mean.

FIVE

How to Rock
Your First 30 Days

- - - - - - - -

Now that you know what is going to kill you, what is deliciously safe, and where you can find everything, let's put it all together, shall we? You may be able to navigate the grocery store in a whole new way, and you're all up to speed on how to dine out without misery, but constantly thinking about where your next meal is coming from and preparing food for yourself are going to be overwhelming. That's why the next 30 days are totally on me.

I'm about to drop a gluten-free meal plan on you for every single day, and most days this will include dessert. Quite frankly, you deserve dessert every day, but before you say "April told me to do it," you might also not want to add "diabetes" to your roster. So take the dessert recipes with a grain of salt (or sugar), and indulge when you feel like you need it, but avoid the bad-for-you stuff when you can. I say this from experience. From an "OhmygodIjustgainedtwenty-pounds!!" experience.

It's really easy to go gluten-free and think you're doing something great for your body (and you are!) only to realize that gluten-free breads, desserts, and snacks are super-duper butt-widening and nap-inducing. I don't want to tempt you to go back to eating gluten just for the weight loss because, as you now know, that could also put you in the hospital. So enjoy your gluten-free food, but remember that gluten-free is not a pass to eat anything else in the entire world that does not contain wheat, barley, rye, or triticale.

Which brings me to the other part of the 30 days that is also going to be challenging. There will be days when no amount of Pumpkin Pound Cake is going to make you feel okay about being gluten-free. You will walk into a restaurant that you thought would be a good fit for your new diet, and the waiter will offer you a plate of lettuce with lemon juice. You might go on a first date and rather drop dead than have to explain your dietary restrictions. I can guarantee that at some point during your first 30 days, some friend or family member will give you guff. Major life changes don't always bring out the best in people, and you're about to find out who is supportive and who would rather you go back to your old, glutenous ways. I want you to know that during this process, you are not alone. There's a whole community of us out there who have been through it, too—feeling hurt, disappointed, left out, and even hopeless.

But it can go both ways. I have been the person crying in a French bakery while her friend won't stop raving about the pastry she's devouring, but I have also been the girl who planned ahead and had the best appetizers at a potluck because I refused to starve at yet another party. And I've been the friend at the table who the waiter flirted with outrageously because his sister was also celiac and he wanted to take care of me. It can go both ways, my friends. You will have great days when everyone "gets it," and you will have horrible days when no one gives a hoot about your well-being. Just like your life was before you had to go gluten-free. I do know for a fact that when I'm well fed, I can deal with the smart-aleck remarks, the lack of understanding from even the most well-meaning restaurant staff, and the jokes made at my expense. And that is why this book is chock-full of recipes—perhaps even more recipes than you'll ever need!—so you can always have a resource when you're hungry and wishing you could just have some decent food already. You're not alone. Have some (gluten-free) cake.

These recipes and plans are representative of what I prepare for myself and my family. Which means most of them are simple and easy to get on the table. Since I do love to cook, and I like to razzle-dazzle on occasion, there are also a few fancy-pants recipes and suggestions in these pages. Save those for the weekend or when you have more time to tinker around in the kitchen. On the nights you come home late and cranky, just grab the gluten-free pasta and take it easy. And remember, you're going to have leftovers, so some of these dishes can stretch into two or three days of meals. (I'm looking at you, enchiladas.) I want to give you gluten-free newbies (and oldies who are trying to expand their gluten-free cooking repertoire) enough options to keep you on the straight-and-narrow gluten-free path.

Of course, these meal plans are only suggestions. Do what makes you happy while you're making a change for your health. It's the only way you'll stick to it and discover the benefits of removing gluten from your diet.

Before you make a grocery list and head off to the store to buy every single thing on these pages, select a handful of recipes to try. Your first trip to the store should be inspiring, so pick what you want to eat and what you know will get you through the first few days. Feel free to flip through the 30 days and pick out your favorites and stick with them for a while if that's what's going to help you get through this drastic dietary change. If what you really want is an entire week of tacos (and I've been there), then load up on corn tortillas and beans and go to town. Don't buy food you're not crazy about when you're just getting started. There's nothing worse than wilting kale staring at you from the crisper. Don't waste time and money on food you won't have time to get to in the next five days.

There are some basics that will really help you out in this transition phase. Consider using this list to stock your kitchen the first time you head out to the grocery store with your new meal plan so that every trip isn't a time-consuming ordeal. Then you can plan on dropping by that organic butcher or farmers' market during the week to get fresh options that go with what you already have at home. While you're picking up your first batch of groceries, stock your pantry with these cook's helpers:

Butter, or ghee if you're dairy-free (ghee is made from milk, but lactose and casein are removed if those are your issues)
All-purpose gluten-free flour
Sea salt
Black pepper

Garlic

Onions

Gluten-free bread/crumbs

Parmesan

Eggs

Rice

Sugar (or sugar substitute)

Brown sugar

Tomatoes or tomato sauce

Olive oil

Vegetable oil

Cinnamon

Vanilla extract

Nutmeg

Red pepper flakes

Ginger, fresh or powdered

Potatoes of any variety

Milk (or milk alternative)

Wheat-free tamari

Wine—white and red (Or perhaps you're more of
a Scotch drinker?)

Don't forget: If you always have some gluten-free
pasta handy, you will never go hungry or panic. You
don't want to wind up at the Wendy's drive-thru at
8 p.m. ordering every baked potato on the menu because your cabinets are empty. That should only happen on your birthday.

A Word on Alcohol

As someone who freaked out when I was first diagnosed
with celiac, I like to say that wine helped me through.
In fact, I just said it a few pages ago! While that's par-

tially true (you can take my dinner rolls, but you can never take my pinot!), the fact is that the alcohol change-up is not that big of a deal when you go gluten-free. Unless you're a beer connoisseur, and then, my friend, you will be sad.

After calling my dietician every time someone told me I couldn't have a gin and tonic, I learned that, really, we gluten-free people can still bend an elbow. As long as it's not Budweiser. There are a lot of rumors out there about vodka, whiskeys, and even wine, but according to my sources (and to Dr. Alessio Fasano in his book, *Gluten Freedom*), we can safely enjoy everything but beer, malt liquor, and a few of those pesky flavored liquors that use barley malt (always check a label!). If you stick to the basics (and the basics don't include beer and malt liquor), you can order from a bar menu with confidence.

The Great GF Booze Debate

I do feel the need to address the many people who have said they have had issues with whiskeys and other spirits, and who believe wine can be contaminated in the barrel. If you're feeling sick after eating or drinking something, stop eating or drinking that thing. We're a sensitive bunch, we're all different, and gluten is not always the culprit when things go awry. If I have more than three cups of coffee in the morning, my stomach will react like I licked a bagel. This doesn't mean that coffee has gluten in it. It does not. My stomach just can't take that extra pressure now that I'm in the celiac club. If you have a shot of bourbon and your gut reacts, stop taking shots of bourbon. Still, bourbon does not contain gluten peptides. That's just science.

(Gluten-Free) Beer Me

With the explosion of gluten-free beers on the market, we aren't really even left out at the kegger. Between the always growing selection of gluten-free beer and the rise in popularity of hard cider, I'd say the gluten-free can drink pretty well. Of course, my advice is always to drink responsibly, not only for the sake of your reputation, safety, and waistline, but also because you can't afford to have altered judgment at the 7-Eleven's snack aisle at 2 a.m.

There are two different kinds of gluten-free beer: those made with alternative grains, such as sorghum, and even vegetables, such as sweet potatoes, and those that remove the gluten after the beer has been made with barley or wheat. Some celiacs and gluten-sensitive people do not want to touch those beers that have even a trace (less than 20 ppm) of gluten after having the gluten removed. I get it. Why tempt fate? No one is going to make you drink those types of gluten-free beers. But I happen to enjoy the flavor of those options because, to me, they taste more like "real" beer. I've never had any ill effects after consuming a beverage (or food) that has less than 20 ppm of gluten. I have, however, had many a negative reaction after being served a meal from a kitchen contaminated with gluten, even though my meal was gluten-free. So while I am incredibly sensitive, the 20 ppm rule that has been approved by many a celiac disease organization holds true for this particular celiac. You may not be able to say the same. So stick to what you know is gluten-free and safe for your belly.

Of course, not drinking alcohol for the 30 days could also be helpful in settling your stomach, joint, skin, sleep, and thinking problems. Alcohol is one of those luxury items, not unlike ice cream, that we celiacs get excited about being able to have even when we have to pass by the donut shop on the way to the ice cream/liquor store. But no one is going to argue that booze and dairy treats are good for your body when you're in a state of upset-edness. Good for your mental well-being? Maybe. But feel free to skip anything that isn't nourishing for your body if you want to focus on wellness and not just the fear of deprivation as you go gluten-free. If you're in a world of hurt from gluten beating down your body, skip the booze, dairy, sugar, and fun. Don't worry, all those crazy good times will still be there when you're back in fighting form and more able to consume food and drink without fear. In fact, whenever I've been brutally gluten-ed, the one thing that helps me get back into shape is removing any and all inflammatory foods from my diet, à la the Whole30 diet (see Resources). Don't punish your already tender body if your skin is just barely healing and you're starting to be able to give up your afternoon nap. Be smart and be healthy.

With that said, I felt it necessary to throw in some really fun gluten-free cocktails during your 30 days to help celebrate your new lifestyle if that's the way you roll. Mix these up at your next party, and no one will notice the mediocre crackers. (And for good gluten-free crackers, see Resources.)

I realize that all this food preparation and cooking information is hard to hear the first time (or the first 20 times), which is why I want to tell you about another option that's popping up all over America. There are places that will actually make you a gluten-free meal or three and deliver them to your home. (See Resources.)

All right, party people, are you ready for 30 days of seriously delicious gluten-free eating, drinking, and being merry? Let's do this!

Five Snacks to Have on Hand When You Just Can't Deal

· · · · ·

The gluten-free are just like everybody else when it comes to not wanting to cook one more meal and not wanting to call and order takeout since you've already eaten in all the good places this week. Sometimes you just need to grab a quick snack and call it a night. Here are five great gluten-free snacks I can turn into mini-meals. I always like to have these ingredients on hand in case I want to skip a big dinner and just get something in my belly.

1. **Mixed nuts.** While I always think having a stash of almonds is great for snacking, I've branched out to mix it up. It's somehow more filling to have a variety of salted, roasted deliciousness instead of only one kind of nut.

2. **Cheese and gluten-free crackers.** The sun does not set on a gluten-free crackerless house in my neighborhood. I always make sure I have a good cheese handy and some crackers when it's time to have appetizers for dinner.

3. **Fruit juice and fresh berries.** You can turn fruit into a thick and filling smoothie by adding juice, a filler like yogurt or sorbet, and lots of ice.

4. **Rice.** Whether it's brown, white, long grain, or short grain, cooking up rice is the quickest way to fill your gluten-free belly. Add milk and sugar for a sweet treat, or throw on wheat-free tamari and some vegetables for a faux stir-fry. But the all-time fave in my house is rice with black beans and cayenne pepper.

5. **Gluten-free pasta.** No matter the variety of gluten-free pasta, you can be eating well in minutes if you boil it up and add butter, Parmesan, and red pepper flakes. If you've got any spare vegetables lying around, steam them and add them to the mix.

SIX

Basic Gluten-Free Cooking Methods and GF Pantry Essentials

· · · · · · ·

Gluten-Free Cooking and Baking Methods

Cooking gluten-free is just like cooking everything else . . . sometimes. To be specific, preparing *naturally* gluten-free foods is not an issue, but once you start experimenting with alternative flours, things can get weird.

I have a few tricks to make your transition much smoother, and your cookies much tastier. The best advice I've ever gotten, and given, is to keep experimenting in the kitchen. Everything will get easier, I promise, and you'll stumble onto some surprisingly delicious methods yourself.

There are some instructions that may cause the casual cook to glaze over while reading. But when you're working with gluten-free recipes, certain practices are crucial for success. Be sure you keep these methods in mind when whipping up your gluten-free meals.

GLUTEN-FREE KITCHEN DO'S

- Always preheat your oven for at least 20 minutes. Gluten-free dough needs a hot oven.
- Always remember to use gluten-free flour for rolling out dough, greasing, and flouring a pan, and any other place where you may be inclined to believe "a little gluten won't hurt." It will. Oh, it will.
- Always chill your cookie dough for at least 30 minutes before shaping and baking.
- Always bring eggs to room temperature before mixing.
- Always test a recipe before you try it out on guests or for holidays. Remember, we're going for *fewer* tears now that we know how to eat safely.
- Always have a gluten-eating friend try your baked goods before sharing with others. Your taste buds will change after not eating gluten for a period of time.
- Always cook with regular olive oil, and make salad dressings and dips with extra virgin olive oil. Regular olive oil withstands heat better, but if you want more flavor, add extra virgin after cooking.
- Always make your own gluten-free dish and bring it to the party. You don't know what else is going on in other people's kitchens.
- Always check your baked goods for doneness with a toothpick or sharp knife. Many gluten-free recipes need more time than a recipe calls for.

- Always eat baked goods quickly, or freeze them. The shelf life of gluten-free homemade baked goods is not as long as the regular ones.

GLUTEN-FREE KITCHEN DON'TS

- Never be afraid to experiment with gluten-free flours. Everything from millet to mesquite is on the market now, so enjoy testing them all in your favorite brownie recipe.
- Never taste the raw dough when using gluten-free flours. You don't want that taste to haunt you, trust me.
- Never toss out a recipe after one failure. Tweak it and try again.
- Never overmix a recipe that uses gluten-free flour.
- Never use the same pots and pans for gluten-free pastas and gluten-filled.
- Never overcook gluten-free pasta. Stop when it's al dente unless you prefer your pasta in a blob.
- Never stop making a recipe you love, even if everyone else hates it. Just don't share.
- Never feel guilty about using premade (gluten-free) cheats in your recipes. Your cooking requirements are hard enough already.

Gluten-Free Pantry Essentials

Setting up your kitchen with gluten-free staples is crucial in making the transition to your new lifestyle simple and stress-free (or stress reducing). Make sure your pantry is stocked with the basics all kitchens should have for easy food preparation. These are my absolute must-haves:

Marinara sauce

Gluten-free pasta

Vanilla extract

Almond extract

Coarse sea salt

Fresh pepper

Frozen gluten-free bread

Olive oil

Extra virgin olive oil

Vegetable oil

Lemons or other citrus fruits

Baking powder

Baking soda

All-purpose gluten-free flour

Gluten-free cornmeal

Eggs

Milk (dairy or alternative)

Variety of cheeses

Corn tortillas

Variety of beans (black, white, pinto, chickpeas)

Rice

Quinoa

Lentils

Herbs, fresh or dried

Butter, unsalted

Sugars (brown, white, turbinado, powdered,
   alternative sugars)

Cornstarch

Red pepper flakes

Gluten-free crackers

Variety of nuts and nut butters

Wheat-free tamari

Hot sauce

Condiments (ketchup, mustard, mayo, GF dressings)

White and red wine vinegar
Fresh fruits
Fresh vegetables
Good dark chocolate

So you're not chopping and sautéing 24/7, give yourself a break with the following premade cheats. Don't forget to make sure they're gluten-free! (See Resources.)

Gluten-Free Cheats

While I'm a big fan of making everything from scratch, I'm also a big fan of not losing my mind. It's true that if we ate like our grandmothers did, we would be much healthier, but my grandmothers did not work 60 hours a week outside the home or have the Internet. (Honestly, that's where our time goes, is it not?) So sometimes we need some help in the form of cheats and prepared foods. I, for one, am not up for making a gluten-free piecrust for every holiday dinner. Luckily, Whole Foods (and others) do that for me. That's what I call a winning cheat. Also, isn't progress *amazing*?

Naturally, when you're purchasing prepared foods, you *must* know what every ingredient is to ensure it is truly gluten-free. The brands I use are gluten-free (see Resources), but you will certainly find other brands at your local grocery stores. Don't forget to read the fine print if you don't want to wind up on the pot.

PREMADE CHEATS

Premade gluten-free pasta
Spray olive oil

Spray canola oil, but make sure it doesn't have added flour

Premade pesto

Frozen rice

Premade polenta (make sure it's GF; not all of them are)

Premade gluten-free piecrust

Marinara sauce

Frozen herbs and garlic

Bagged, prewashed greens

Gluten-free pancake and waffle mix

Gluten-free baguettes

Gluten-free cheese bread

Gluten-free waffles

Precooked lentils and beans

BBQ sauce

Ranch dressing

Now you've got to make all of this stuff work together. While I love having a dough cutter, a stand mixer, and other one-trick-pony gadgets (pizza scissors, anyone?), you really can get by with the basics. Of course, I call an ice cream maker a basic, just so you know. Still, I firmly believe these are the tools you'll need to mix, match, and maximize your gluten-free kitchen.

KITCHEN TOOLS

Large roasting pan

2 (9-by-13-inch) baking pans

3 (8- or 9-inch) cake rounds

Loaf pan

3 skillets: small, medium, and large

1 cast-iron skillet

3 saucepans: small, medium, and large

2 baking sheets

2 muffin tins

2 metal whisks

2 strainers, one large and one small

3 casserole dishes in varying sizes

6 mixing bowls in varying sizes

Measuring spoons in all denominations

Measuring cups in all denominations

Liquid measuring cup

Meat tenderizer

Pizza pan

Box grater

Hand grater

Microplane

Corkscrew

Can opener

Meat thermometer

Candy thermometer

Salad spinner

Kitchen shears

Hand juicer

Blender or food processor

Hand masher

Vegetable peeler

Full set of knives (including bread knife)

Knife sharpener

Sifter

Hand mixer

2 plastic spatulas, 1 metal spatula

2 large mixing spoons

2 to 4 serving spoons

Salad bowl

Full set of dishes
Ladle
Tongs
Slotted spoon
Timer
Toaster oven

Help! I'm Surrounded by Gluten-Free Flour!

One of the first things people want to know about when they go gluten-free is what's up with all those crazy flours? It's true, there are some crazy gluten-free flours out there. Mostly because there have been some desperate gluten intolerants in the world trying to re-create their favorite dinner rolls. Necessity has never been the mother of invention more than when a celiac craves a flaky crust.

While most of the time I'll pick an all-purpose gluten-free flour that does not require any gums (more on gums later), you should experiment with a variety of grain flours that are safe for the gluten-free and see what you like best. Here's how they break down:

ALTERNATIVE GRAIN FLOURS

Sorghum flour
Almond flour (a fave)
Hazelnut flour
Walnut flour
Coconut flour (another fave)
Rice flour (white, sweet, and brown)
Tapioca flour
Garbanzo bean flour

Potato flour

Soy flour

Buckwheat (yet another favorite)

Amaranth flour

Millet flour (great for making a roux)

Teff flour

Cornmeal (has to be labeled gluten-free)

And the new kids on the block:

Mesquite flour (mostly for adding a cinnamon
  flavor)

Green banana flour

So how do you replace that sticky gluten? While using xanthan and guar gums in very small amounts have historically been a go-to in gluten-free baking, a lot of us in this field are starting to experiment without these thickening and binding agents. Some people find xanthan and guar gums difficult to digest, and others just don't like having any additives in their food. Personally, I've left them out a few times when I was cooking and found I didn't notice a difference. Some recipes will need the stability (think fluffy popovers), but others, like a standard chocolate cake, can probably do without. Note: All-purpose gluten-free flours generally have xanthan gum added into the mix, so you wouldn't add any to your recipe if you're using one of those brands.

Gluten-free starches and binding agents include:

Xanthan gum

Guar gum

Arrowroot

Tapioca starch
Potato starch
Cornstarch

A lot of cooks create their own all-purpose blends using these ingredients. You can follow some great recipes from these chefs, or you can purchase an all-purpose gluten-free flour in the store. (See Resources.)

Having plenty of substitutes for your gluten-filled flour is a great idea in case you have a sudden urge to make fried chicken. At the same time, cooking with naturally gluten-free food will feel much more satisfying in the long run. Plus, you won't have to experiment since you're already familiar with how an omelet should look and taste. You can stop stressing out about measurements and liquids if your world-famous vanilla bean ice cream is on the menu. It's just easier to skip the cookies altogether, but hey, I know we all need them sometimes.

So now you know how to have rockin' success in your gluten-free kitchen. Take a deep breath, because that's a lot to remember. (Keep this book handy in your kitchen until it becomes second nature.)

SEVEN

Your 30-Day Meal Plan

．．．．．．．

Welcome to the first day of the rest of your gluten-free life. First of all, I would like to express mad sympathy. Second, I would like to offer you a martini because, guess what? It's gluten-free.

My hope is that you find yourself surprised by the wide variety of foods you can eat that are naturally gluten-free or easily converted into a gluten-free dish. Once you're at the end of these 30 days of gluten-free eating, you're going to be an expert on pulling together a delicious lunch for work or even a dinner party.

So let's get started with the first day of your 30-day gluten-free meal plan! Remember, you can mix and match if you're not feeling like chicken, booze, or dessert all in one day. Use this plan as a guide to get you through 30 delicious days to a new way of eating—a way of eating that will make you feel so much better

you won't even know why you used to love brioche.
Probably.

•DAY 1•

Breakfast: Huevos Rancheros

Lunch: Grilled Cheese and Bacon,* Sweet Potato
  Chips

Dinner: Asian Pork Chops,* Brussels Sprouts with
  Pistachios

Cocktail: Lillet Blanc Martini

Dessert: Chocolate fudge sundae

* Make your day vegetarian: Drop the bacon at lunch; have
some gluten-free pasta with red sauce instead of pork chops
for dinner.

•DAY 2•

Breakfast: Gluten-free pancakes

Lunch: Cuban-Style White Rice and Black Beans

Snack: Almond butter on celery sticks

Dinner: Sesame-Crusted Tuna Steak, Dill
  Asparagus

•DAY 3•
YOU'RE GOING OUT TO DINNER!!!

Breakfast: Sweet Potato Hash Browns and
  eggs

Lunch: Blackened Salmon Salad

Dinner: You want to head to your local Mexican joint. Mostly because it's easy to order gluten-free there, and I want your first dining-out experience to be positive. Please note: If you live in Texas, avoid the Tex-Mex places unless you want to cry into your chimichanga. Best options to order include:

Enchiladas

Hard-shell tacos

Nachos

Fajitas with corn tortillas

Margaritas!

•DAY 4•

Breakfast: World's Greatest Granola

Lunch: Classic Tuna Melt

Snack: Melon Balls of Fun

Dinner: Mesclun Salad with Goat Cheese Croquettes, Smoky-Sweet Potato Soup

•DAY 5•

To start your day right, chop up about a tablespoon of chives, chervil, and thyme, and beat with two eggs. Scramble them up and enjoy.

Breakfast: Herbed Scrambled Eggs

Lunch: BBQ Chicken Salad,* Strawberry Lemonade

Dinner: Cheesy Quinoa Broccoli Mac

Dessert: Brownies with Pumpkin Bourbon
  Sauce

* Have a vegetarian day by substituting tofu for the chicken
in the salad. Use a BBQ sauce that doesn't contain bacon,
and you're all set.

• **D A Y 6** •

Breakfast: Almond Scone, fresh berries

Lunch: Veggie Soba Noodles

Snack: Go nuts! Grab a bag of mixed nuts, salt
  them up, and dig in.

Cocktail: Limoncello

Dinner: Crispy Pork Loin,* Sweet Potato Hash
  Browns

* Substitute quinoa leftovers for a vegetarian option.

• **D A Y 7** •

You didn't eat all those scones yet, right? If you did,
make another batch.

Breakfast: Almond Scone, melon

Lunch: Steak and Spinach Salad

Snack: GF crackers and nut butter

Dinner: Spicy Black Bean Enchiladas,
  Green Rice

Dessert: Chocolate Beet Bundt Cake

•DAY 8•

Breakfast: Biscuit breakfast sandwich (GF biscuit, scrambled eggs, cheddar cheese, and bacon)

Lunch: Persian Rice, simple side salad

Snack: Chocolate Beet Bundt Cake

Dinner: Spicy Meatloaf, roasted broccoli

•DAY 9•

Breakfast: World's Greatest Granola

Lunch: Leftovers! Meatloaf, enchiladas, whatever makes you happy

Dinner: Cheesy Cauliflower Pizza

Cocktail: Grab a gluten-free beer. (See Resources.)

Dessert: Buckeyes

•DAY 10•

Breakfast: Canadian Bacon Eggs Benedict

Lunch: Chicken Parmesan

Snack: Cheese and Chive Crackers

Dinner: Porchetta, roasted winter squash

•DAY 11•

Breakfast: GF Rice Chex with fresh berries

Lunch: Porchetta sandwich

Snack: Crab Cakes

Dinner: Veggie Soba Noodles

•DAY 12•

Breakfast: Breakfast Pizza

Lunch: Rich Mushroom Risotto

Snack: Cheese and Chive Crackers

Dinner: Chicken Mole with Rice

•DAY 13•

Breakfast: Leek and Bacon Quiche

Lunch: Mesclun Salad with Goat Cheese Croquettes

Snack: Fresh fruit

Dinner: Chicken Piccata with Spaghetti

•DAY 14•

Breakfast: World's Greatest Granola

Lunch: Lentil and Lox Salad

Dinner: Skirt Steak with Chimichurri Sauce, Dill
Asparagus

Cocktail: It's wine o'clock

Dessert: Lemon-Raspberry Ice

•DAY 15•

Breakfast: Herbed Scrambled Eggs (see page 83)
with melon

Lunch: Pernil tacos

Snack: Cheesy Bacon Kale Chips

Dinner: Turkey Ragout with GF pasta

• DAY 16 •

Breakfast: Warm quinoa with almond milk and honey

Lunch: BBQ Chicken Strips

Snack: Almond butter and GF crackers

Dinner: Fish and Chips

• DAY 17 •

Breakfast: Melon Balls of Fun, yogurt

Lunch: (With a dinner like this, you'd better just eat lettuce—kidding!) Quinoa Bowl

Snack: Spiced Almonds

Dinner: Truffle Cheeseburgers, Smashed Potatoes with Bacon

Dessert: Caramel Popcorn Sundae

• DAY 18 •

Breakfast: Sweet Potato Hash Browns

Lunch: Polenta Torta

Dinner: Kung Pao Pork, P.F. Chang's Asian Lettuce Wraps

Cocktail: Hibiscus Gimlet

Dessert: Lemon Bars

•DAY 19•

Breakfast: Gluten-free oatmeal with honey

Lunch: Polenta Torta

Snack: KIND Bar

Dinner: Cheesy Cauliflower Pizza

•DAY 20•

Breakfast: Ham and Cheese Waffle

Lunch: Cuban-Style Black Beans and White Rice

Snack: Baked Brie with Apples and GF crackers

Dinner: Tuna Tartare and green salad

•DAY 21•

Breakfast: Almond Scone

Lunch: Quinoa Bowl

Dinner: Spinach Enchiladas

Cocktail: Jalapeño Margarita

Dessert: Sugar Cookie Cheesecake

•DAY 22•

Breakfast: GF Chex (Rice, Corn, or go crazy with Chocolate)

Lunch: Spinach Enchilada leftovers

Appetizer: Polenta Crostini with White Beans and Kale

Dinner: Bacon-Wrapped Scallops

•DAY 23•

Breakfast: Bob's Red Mill Mighty Tasty Hot Cereal

Lunch: Easy BBQ Pulled Pork sandwich

Snack: Popcorn with sea salt

Dinner: Chicken Masala-ish and GF naan bread

•DAY 24•

Breakfast: Canadian Bacon Eggs Benedict

Lunch: Easy Chicken Soup with Rice

Snack: Kale and Artichoke Dip

Dinner: London Broil, Twice-Baked Potatoes

•DAY 25•

Breakfast: Sweet Potato Hash Browns and eggs

Lunch: Blackened Salmon Salad

Dinner: Coconut Flour Tortilla

Cocktail: Jalapeño Margarita

Dessert: Cheesecake Ice Cream

•DAY 26•

Breakfast: GF oatmeal with honey

Lunch: Zucchini Pasta and Meatballs

Snack: Deep-Fried Chocolate Cream Cookies

Dinner: Asian Pork Chops, Brussels Sprouts with Pistachios

•DAY 27•

Breakfast: GF buttermilk pancakes

Lunch: Grilled Cheese and Bacon, Sweet Potato Chips

Snack: Melon Balls of Fun

Dinner: Pernil tacos and Green Rice

•DAY 28•

Breakfast: Herbed Scrambled Eggs (see page 83)

Lunch: Cuban-Style White Rice and Black Beans

Dinner: Fish and Chips

Cocktail: Grab a cider, you deserve it!

Dessert: Bourbon Joe Cake

•DAY 29•

Breakfast: Canadian Bacon Eggs Benedict

Lunch: BBQ Chicken Salad

Snack: Spiced Almonds

Dinner: Spaghetti Squash with Pesto

•DAY 30•

Breakfast: Warm rice with honey and milk

Lunch: Classic Tuna Melt

Dinner: Skirt Steak with Chimichurri Sauce, Twice-Baked Potatoes

Cocktail: The Perfect G&T

Dessert: Mini Ice Cream Pecan Balls

You did it!! Now, wasn't that delicious? Make a note of your favorites, and those will be your new go-to meals when you're feeling deprived. Congratulations, you're a gluten-free gourmand.

EIGHT

Recipes, Recipes, Recipes

· · · · · · ·

· · · · · · ·

LEEK AND BACON QUICHE

If you have mastered a gluten-free piecrust, congratulations! Personally, I find it an exercise in frustration, so I start with a premade piecrust for this delicious breakfast dish. Watch out if you reheat it and take it to work—the amazing aroma will make you the most popular gluten-free worker in the cubicle.

PREP TIME: 10 minutes
COOK TIME: 1 hour

> *premade gluten-free piecrust*
> *8 ounces bacon, cubed*
> *2 leeks, cut into thin slices*
> *1 teaspoon chopped thyme*
> *salt and pepper*
> *5 ounces Gruyère, grated*
> *3 eggs*
> *2 egg yolks*
> *2 cups half-and-half*

1. Preheat oven to 375 degrees.
2. Thaw gluten-free piecrust for at least 1 hour. You can also pop it into a hot oven for 10 minutes to get that extra crisp feel. While crust is warming up, cook bacon in large skillet over medium-high heat until crispy. Remove bacon and drain, keeping 1 teaspoon bacon grease in skillet.
3. Cook leeks and thyme in same skillet with bacon grease. Add salt and pepper, and cook until leeks are slightly brown, 5 to 7 minutes.
4. Combine Gruyère, leek mixture, and bacon in medium bowl.
5. Whisk eggs, egg yolks, and half-and-half together in separate medium bowl. Add pinch of salt and pepper.

6. Spoon cheese, leek, and bacon mixture into gluten-free piecrust. Pour egg mixture over top and bake for 40 minutes, or until center is firm.

MAKES: 8 servings

· · · · · · · ·

SWEET POTATO HASH BROWNS

This incredibly easy dish has turned into my favorite breakfast. You can prep with one potato for an entire week and just fry a little up each morning. I like it by itself, with a fried egg, or even with some sausage and kale. It's the base for a fantastic start to your day.

PREP TIME: 8 minutes
COOK TIME: 8 minutes

> 1 large sweet potato
> 1 teaspoon sea salt
> 1 teaspoon red pepper flakes
> 1 tablespoon olive oil

1. Using a box grater, grate entire sweet potato into medium bowl. Toss with sea salt and red pepper flakes, evenly distributing spices.
2. Heat olive oil in medium skillet on medium-high.
3. Using a ¼ measuring cup, scoop sweet potato into rounds and cook for 3 to 4 minutes per side, until brown and crispy. Remove from skillet and drain on paper towel–covered plate.
4. Serve alone or with sausage or a fried egg.

MAKES: 6 servings

· · · · · · ·

BREAKFAST PIZZA

Pizza for breakfast will be exciting for the kids, but as a full-grown lady, I admit to being excited by this fun breakfast as well. Choose your toppings, and mix and match any way you like. Make two or three versions when you have overnight guests and you'll be the coolest host ever.

PREP TIME: 15 minutes
COOK TIME: 15 minutes

> 1 box gluten-free pizza crust mix or 1 premade gluten-free pizza crust
> ½ cup marinara sauce
> 5 eggs
> 2 sausage links, cooked and crumbled
> ½ cup cheddar cheese, grated

1. Preheat oven to 450 degrees. Prepare gluten-free pizza crust mix as instructions direct and roll out onto pizza pan.
2. Make 5 indentations in pizza dough for eggs. Cover pizza dough with marinara sauce.
3. Crack each egg into a well and allow to settle. Cover rest of pizza with sausage, then top with grated cheese.
4. Bake for 15 minutes or until edges are brown and crispy. Remove from oven and allow to cool 2 to 3 minutes before slicing and serving.

MAKES: 8 servings

· · · · · · ·

ALMOND SCONES

Scones are basically fancy biscuits. While you can add in any mixes you like, I'm a fan of using the almond meal and sliced almonds. Yes, it's almazing (sorry).

PREP TIME: 15 minutes
COOK TIME: 10–15 minutes

> 1½ cups all-purpose gluten-free flour + more
>   for rolling
> 1 tablespoon baking powder
> ½ cup almond meal
> ¼ teaspoon sea salt
> ½ stick butter
> 1 teaspoon vanilla extract
> 1 tablespoon maple syrup
> ¾ cup milk + 2 tablespoons for brushing
> ½ cup thinly sliced almonds
> ¼ cup sugar

1. Preheat oven to 450 degrees. Line baking tray with parchment paper.
2. In large bowl, combine flour, baking powder, almond meal, and sea salt. Using pastry cutter, cut butter into dough.
3. Add vanilla and maple syrup, and slowly pour milk in and mix until just combined.
4. Cover hard surface with flour and flour your rolling pin to roll out dough into a circle. Cut dough into 4 triangles and transfer to baking sheet.

5. Brush tops of scones with milk and sprinkle sliced almonds evenly over scones. Sprinkle sugar and bake for 10 to 15 minutes until golden brown. Remove from heat and serve warm.

MAKES: 4 servings

· · · · · · · ·

HUEVOS RANCHEROS

This classic Mexican breakfast dish is not only easy (especially if you make the beans the night before) but a crowd pleaser. Cotija cheese is my favorite for most Mexican dishes, but if you can't find it, grab some Monterey Jack or cheddar cheese and go to town.

PREP TIME: 15 minutes
COOK TIME: 30 minutes, or 10 minutes if beans are made ahead of time

> *1 tablespoon olive oil*
> *1 clove garlic, diced*
> *½ cup black beans*
> *¼ teaspoon cumin*
> *½ teaspoon hot sauce*
> *salt and pepper*
> *4 eggs*
> *4 gluten-free corn tortillas*
> *1 avocado, sliced*
> *4 tablespoons salsa*
> *cotija cheese, crumbled*

1. You can prepare beans the night before to save time. Just reheat in microwave or on stovetop. To prepare

beans, heat olive oil in small saucepan and add garlic. Cook for 1 to 2 minutes until garlic is soft. Add black beans, and season with cumin, hot sauce, and salt and pepper. If beans don't have any liquid reserves, add ⅛ cup of water at this time. Allow to cook for 15 minutes on medium-low.

2. Fry 4 eggs sunny-side up by spraying pan with olive oil cooking spray and heating on medium for 1 minute. Crack egg into pan and allow egg to get crisp on the edges, but center should still be movable.

3. While you're frying your eggs, heat each tortilla for 1 minute per side on dry skillet over medium heat.

4. Assemble huevos rancheros by spooning beans onto each tortilla, topping beans with a fried egg, adding a slice of avocado, then topping with salsa and cotija cheese.

MAKES: 4 servings

• • • • • • • •

BREAKFAST STRATA

Though most traditional breakfast strata recipes call for the bread and other ingredients to be layered over and over, that doesn't quite work with gluten-free bread since it's not as absorbent as regular bread. If you layer more than as directed here (bread, vegetables on top of the bread, bacon crumbled over vegetables, and egg mixture poured over the top), you'll need to increase the cook time and will risk burning the vegetables on top. A gluten-free strata won't have all the volume of a regular strata, but it will still have all the taste.

PREP TIME: 25 minutes
COOK TIME: 15 to 20 minutes

> 1 gluten-free baguette
> ½ cup sliced mushrooms
> ¼ cup finely diced yellow onion
> 2 to 3 slices bacon, cooked and crumbled
> 1 cup broccoli florets, chopped
> 1½ tablespoons fresh flat leaf parsley, finely chopped
> juice of ½ lemon (or more to taste)
> 4 large eggs
> ¼ cup milk
> ¾ teaspoon kosher salt
> 1½ teaspoons Italian seasoning

1. Preheat oven to 350 degrees.
2. Slice gluten-free baguette into ½-inch pieces and set aside.
3. Slice mushrooms until you have ½ cup (about 3 to 4 medium-sized mushrooms) and finely dice yellow onion until you have ¼ cup (about ¼-inch slice of onion).
4. Cook bacon over medium heat. When bacon is cooked to your liking, transfer it to a dish and crumble, but leave bacon fat in pan. Add mushrooms and onion to pan with bacon fat and cook over medium-low heat until soft. Remove from heat.
5. Steam broccoli florets until fork tender. Transfer to a bowl or large measuring cup.
6. Add mushrooms and onion to bowl with broccoli, and add parsley. Squeeze lemon juice over top and stir to incorporate.
7. Spray bottom of 8-by-10-inch casserole dish with

gluten-free cooking spray or coconut oil spray. Tear baguette slices into 2 to 3 pieces each and layer in bottom of casserole dish. Layer broccoli, mushroom, and onion mixture over top, and tuck some of the vegetables into crevices where they can fit between bread chunks. Sprinkle crumbled bacon on top of vegetables.

8. Beat eggs with milk, salt, and Italian seasoning. Pour over top of bread and vegetables in casserole dish, distributing evenly.

9. Bake for 15 to 20 minutes or until egg is completely cooked through. Remove from oven, allow to cool slightly, and slice and serve.

MAKES: 2 large or 4 small servings

• • • • • • • •

WORLD'S GREATEST GRANOLA

You're getting all kinds of goodness that is also good for you in this amazing gluten-free granola recipe. Raw cacao powder (rather than regular cocoa powder) makes all the difference in this recipe. Regular Dutch-process cocoa powder is not an equivalent substitute because it will result in the granola tasting too bitter.

PREP TIME: 20 minutes
COOK TIME: 45 minutes

WET

4 tablespoons brown rice syrup
2 tablespoons raw blue agave syrup
4 tablespoons unsweetened applesauce

½ cup coconut sugar

3 tablespoons coconut oil

DRY

3 cups gluten-free rolled oats

1½ tablespoons chia seeds

1 tablespoon instant coffee

1 teaspoon ground cinnamon

1 tablespoon raw cacao powder

3 tablespoons hemp seeds

2 tablespoons light brown flax seeds

½ cup popped amaranth

1 teaspoon kosher salt

1. Preheat oven to 300 degrees.
2. In saucepan over medium heat, add all wet ingredients and stir well. Bring to boil, stirring frequently, then reduce to simmer for about 5 to 7 minutes. Continue to stir frequently.
3. In deep bowl or pot, add all dry ingredients and stir to mix well.
4. Add warm wet mixture to dry mixture and stir to coat everything.
5. Spread coated granola on parchment-lined baking sheet and bake for 45 minutes on middle rack. Remove pan from oven briefly to stir every 15 minutes to be sure it bakes evenly.
6. As granola cools, it will stiffen. You can break up the pieces once it's cooled.
7. Store in airtight container for up to 4 weeks.

MAKES: 1½ pounds of granola

·······

HAM AND CHEESE WAFFLES

This is my new favorite weekend treat. I mean, ham and cheese in waffles? Yes, please. It's a very Southern recipe, but people from all over the place will dig in.

PREP TIME: 10 minutes
COOK TIME: 5 minutes per waffle

> *2 eggs*
> *1¾ cups milk*
> *½ cup vegetable oil*
> *2 tablespoons honey*
> *½ teaspoon vanilla extract*
> *2 cups all-purpose gluten-free flour*
> *4 teaspoons baking powder*
> *1 cup cheddar cheese, grated*
> *1 cup diced ham*
> *maple syrup*

1. Spray waffle iron with gluten-free cooking spray and preheat.
2. Beat eggs in large bowl until fluffy. Add milk, vegetable oil, honey, and vanilla. Whisk in flour 1 cup at a time. Add baking powder and combine completely. Mix cheddar cheese and ham into waffle batter.
3. Pour 1 cup into standard waffle iron (more if your iron is larger) and cook according to manufacturer's directions. Clean melted cheese off iron between waffles if necessary.

4. Store cooked waffles in 200-degree oven to keep warm if not serving immediately.
5. Serve with maple syrup.

MAKES: 6 servings

· · · · · · ·

CANADIAN BACON EGGS BENEDICT

This fancy breakfast becomes gluten-free by swapping out your traditional English muffin for a gluten-free version. Again, you can make these from scratch, but it's *so* much easier if you pick up a package from your grocer's freezer. One tip: When you're making the hollandaise sauce, be sure you don't allow the boiling water in the lower pot to touch the upper pan or bowl when you're whisking. It will turn that egg into a scramble.

PREP TIME: 20 minutes
COOK TIME: 10 minutes

HOLLANDAISE SAUCE

4 egg yolks
1 tablespoon fresh lemon juice
1 stick butter, melted and cooled
⅛ teaspoon cayenne
⅛ teaspoon sea salt
⅛ teaspoon freshly ground black pepper

EGGS

2 gluten-free English muffins, separated
4 slices Canadian bacon

2 quarts water
1 tablespoon fresh lemon juice
4 large eggs

1. Boil water in bottom of double boiler or small saucepan.
2. In top part of double boiler or in stainless steel bowl, rapidly whisk egg yolks and lemon juice together until mixture begins to thicken. Place egg mixture over boiling water without pan or bowl touching water and add melted butter while continuing to whisk rapidly.
3. After egg mixture has doubled in size, remove from heat. Add cayenne, salt, and pepper and mix well. Set aside.
4. Place your gluten-free English muffins into toaster and brown to desired crustiness.
5. Place Canadian bacon slices in medium skillet and cook on medium heat for 3 to 4 minutes, flipping over once.
6. Boil 2 quarts water in large, shallow saucepan. After water is rapidly boiling, turn heat down to low and maintain simmer.
7. Add lemon juice to water immediately before slipping each egg into water gently so it does not break. If your pan isn't large enough for 4 eggs, cook 2 at a time. Cook eggs on simmer for 3 minutes or until egg white is white and yolk is bright. Remove immediately and serve on gluten-free English muffin topped with Canadian bacon.
8. Ladle hollandaise sauce on top and serve.

MAKES: 4 servings

• A P P E T I Z E R S   A N D   S N A C K S •

Kale and Artichoke Dip
Sweet Potato Chips
Spiced Almonds
Melon Balls of Fun
Cheese and Chive Crackers
Baked Brie with Apples
Cheesy Bacon Kale Chips
Tuna Tartare
Polenta Crostini with White Beans and Kale

. . . .

KALE AND ARTICHOKE DIP

This is one of those apps that will go fast, with no
leftovers. To make it as guest-friendly as possible, be
sure you chop your kale into small pieces, as no one
should have to chew dip.

PREP TIME: 15 minutes
COOK TIME: 15 minutes

4 ounces cream cheese, at room temperature
½ cup Gruyère, shredded
¼ cup Parmesan, grated, + 2 teaspoons for
covering dish
½ cup half-and-half
½ bunch kale, deveined and chopped
½ cup artichoke hearts, chopped (if buying
canned, squeeze liquid out and allow
to dry)
1 clove garlic, minced
½ teaspoon salt

½ teaspoon gluten-free Worcestershire sauce
¼ teaspoon freshly ground black pepper

1. Preheat oven to 375 degrees.
2. Combine cream cheese, Gruyère, Parmesan, and half-and-half in large saucepan over medium heat, stirring until combined.
3. Stir in kale, artichoke hearts, and garlic, and heat for 5 minutes. Add salt, Worcestershire sauce, and pepper, and remove from heat.
4. Transfer ingredients into pie pan or small baking dish and sprinkle Parmesan on top. Bake for 15 minutes or until top is slightly golden brown. Serve with crudités or gluten-free crackers.

MAKES: 8 servings

• • • • • • •

SWEET POTATO CHIPS

When you're making your own healthier version of chips, feel free to create Paleo-friendly "nachos" by adding beef chili and guacamole on top. Or, you know, just eat them all while sitting in front of the TV. Either way.

PREP TIME: 5 minutes
COOK TIME: 8 minutes per batch

1 quart vegetable oil
2 large sweet potatoes
salt
freshly ground black pepper
paprika

1. Fill deep fryer with vegetable oil or pour enough oil into deep skillet to cover sweet potato slices. Preheat fryer on high (if using skillet, heat oil over medium-high heat).
2. Leaving skin on, thinly slice sweet potatoes using mandolin or very sharp knife.
3. Place handfuls of potato slices in oil and fry until crispy, 5 to 8 minutes. If you're using a skillet, turn potato slices after 3 minutes to fry opposite side.
4. Remove chips from oil, and drain on paper towel–covered plate to absorb excess oil. Transfer chips to serving basket and sprinkle with salt, pepper, and paprika to taste.

MAKES: 8 servings

•••••••

SPICED ALMONDS

Be sure to use blanched almonds in this recipe to allow the spices to really soak in and give it that punch. This also makes a great holiday gift that's healthy, delicious, and, of course, gluten-free.

PREP TIME: 5 minutes
COOK TIME: 20 minutes

1 egg white
1 teaspoon freshly squeezed
   lime juice
¼ teaspoon cumin
¼ teaspoon chili powder
¼ teaspoon salt
¼ teaspoon paprika

¼ teaspoon black pepper
2 cups blanched almonds

1. Preheat oven to 350 degrees.
2. Beat egg white in medium bowl. Add lime juice, then add spices and mix thoroughly. Add almonds to mixture and coat evenly.
3. Spread almonds on baking sheet covered in parchment paper and bake for 20 minutes.
4. Remove almonds from oven and allow to cool. Break apart to serve.

MAKES: 6 servings

. . . .

MELON BALLS OF FUN

This makes a perfect snack for kids by turning regular old fruit into balls they can pop right in their mouths. Somehow fruit tastes better when it's in a fun shape, right?

PREP TIME: 10 minutes

1 honeydew melon
1 cantaloupe
½ watermelon
1 teaspoon lemon juice
2 teaspoons fresh mint, finely chopped

1. Cut honeydew melon and cantaloupe in half and remove seeds.
2. Using melon baller or small ice cream scoop (melon baller preferred), scoop out balls of honeydew, can-

taloupe, and watermelon, and transfer to large bowl. Toss and mix.

3. Pour lemon juice over melon balls and toss again.
4. Sprinkle mint on top of melon balls and serve.

MAKES: 16 servings

· · · · · · ·

CHEESE AND CHIVE CRACKERS

You don't always want to make homemade gluten-free crackers, but these flavorful and easy snacks are a good time. Be sure to leave very few holes when you roll out the dough, so that the crackers stay together. These crackers are also addictive, so be sure you have plenty of time to dedicate to cracker eating once you've made them.

PREP TIME: 15 minutes + 30 minutes chill time
COOK TIME: 15 minutes

3 tablespoons butter, softened
1 cup shredded Fontina
1 tablespoon minced chives
½ cup all-purpose gluten-free flour
dash of salt
½ teaspoon pepper

1. In a medium bowl, beat butter until fluffy. Add Fontina, chives, flour, salt, and pepper.
2. Transfer mixture to parchment paper and roll into a log. Refrigerate for 30 minutes.
3. Preheat oven to 375 degrees.
4. Slice log into ¼-inch slices and place on lightly

greased baking sheet. Bake for 15 minutes or until crispy and brown.

5. Serve with your favorite cheese or dip, or enjoy plain.

MAKES: 10 servings

• • • • • • •

BAKED BRIE WITH APPLES

An easy way to impress your guests, this dish looks incredibly fancy while being ridiculously easy to make. I'll be honest, I sometimes skip the apples and just eat the delicious melted cheese. You do what you feel is right.

PREP TIME: 5 minutes
COOK TIME: 10 minutes

1 medium Brie wheel
3 tablespoons honey or jam
1 green apple, sliced

1. Preheat oven to 350 degrees.
2. Leaving rind intact, place Brie wheel in ceramic baking dish and cover with honey or jam of your choice. Bake Brie for 10 minutes.
3. Remove from oven and allow Brie to cool for 10 minutes.
4. Serve with apple slices and gluten-free crackers.

MAKES: 8 servings

· · · · · · · ·

CHEESY BACON KALE CHIPS

Kale chips have grown in popularity for all ages, but for those who aren't quite convinced, just add some bacon and nutritional yeast. That'll do it! Of course, you can make this vegetarian by skipping the bacon and substituting olive oil.

PREP TIME: 8 minutes
COOK TIME: 20 minutes

> *3 slices bacon*
> *1 head kale, deveined and chopped*
> *1 tablespoon nutritional yeast*
> *salt and pepper*

1. Preheat oven to 300 degrees.
2. Cook bacon slices until crispy, reserving bacon drippings. Allow bacon drippings to cool for about 10 minutes.
3. Chop kale into bite-size pieces and place on large baking sheet. Pour drippings over kale and evenly distribute nutritional yeast as well. Add salt and pepper, and bake kale for 20 minutes or until crispy.
4. While kale chips are cooking, crumble bacon into bits.
5. Remove kale chips from oven and transfer to bowl. Sprinkle bacon bits over kale chips and serve.

MAKES: 6 servings

·······

TUNA TARTARE

I was determined to re-create a gluten-free version of the best tuna tartare I've ever had from one of my favorite restaurants in New York, North Square. While the presentation may not be as beautiful, it still tastes pretty darned amazing.

PREP TIME: 10 minutes

> ½ pound tuna steak, sashimi grade
> 2 tablespoons extra virgin olive oil
> ⅛ teaspoon wheat-free tamari
> ¼ teaspoon sea salt
> ½ teaspoon freshly ground black pepper
> 1½ teaspoons capers
> 1 avocado, cubed
> 2 tablespoons fresh lemon juice
> ½ teaspoon sesame seeds, toasted

1. Using sharp knife, cutting with the grain, cut tuna steak into cubes and place in small serving bowl.
2. Add extra virgin olive oil, wheat-free tamari, sea salt, and pepper to tuna and stir well.
3. Add capers—with or without brine, to your taste—to tuna mixture and combine. Add avocado and cover with fresh lemon juice.
4. Sprinkle with toasted sesame seeds and serve with gluten-free bagel chips or gluten-free crackers.

MAKES: 4 servings

· · · · · · ·

POLENTA CROSTINI WITH WHITE BEANS AND KALE

Be sure you buy gluten-free polenta, as some cornmeal-based foods do have flour added. Turn this delicious appetizer into a side dish by skipping the polenta and serving up the white beans and kale solo.

PREP TIME: 10 minutes
COOK TIME: 30 minutes

> 1 (18-ounce) package precooked gluten-free polenta
> 1 tablespoon olive oil
> 1 clove garlic, minced
> 1 head kale, deveined and chopped
> 1 cup white beans, canned
> 1 teaspoon red pepper flakes
> salt and pepper

1. Preheat oven to 350 degrees.
2. Lightly spray large baking sheet with olive oil spray.
3. Slice polenta into ½-inch circles and place on baking sheet. Bake for 10 to 15 minutes or until light golden brown.
4. While polenta is crisping, add olive oil to medium skillet and heat on medium-high for 3 minutes. Turn heat down to medium, add garlic, and cook until slightly softened, about 3 minutes.
5. Add chopped kale to skillet and cover generously with olive oil and garlic. Cook until wilted, 3 to 5 minutes.

6. Add white beans with about 1 teaspoon of bean liquid from can, red pepper flakes, salt, and pepper to kale, and combine. Cook for another 3 minutes or until fully warm.

7. Remove polenta from oven and plate. Add 1 to 2 tablespoons of kale and white bean mixture to each polenta round.

MAKES: 12 servings

·MAIN COURSES AND SIDES·

Easy Chicken Soup with Rice

Spinach Enchiladas

Truffle Cheeseburgers

Sunday Chicken

London Broil

Cuban-Style White Rice and Black Beans

Kale, Chicken, and Goat Cheese Salad

Veggie Soba Noodles

Amy's Best Pasta Ever

Chicken Parmesan

Wilted Greens

Polenta Torta

Cheesy Cauliflower Pizza

BBQ Spare Ribs

Pan-Seared Halibut

Spaghetti Squash with Pesto

Spicy Black Bean Enchiladas

Lentil and Lox Salad

Bacon-Wrapped Scallops

Smashed Potatoes with Bacon

Steak and Spinach Salad

Twice-Baked Potatoes

• The Gluten-Free Cheat Sheet •

Parmesan Popovers
Spicy Tofu Stir-Fry
Chicken Masala-ish
Smoky-Sweet Potato Soup
Chicken Mole with Rice
Spicy Meatloaf
Crispy Pork Loin
Mesclun Salad with Goat Cheese Croquettes
Sweet and Sour Chicken
Arugula, Corn, and Red Onion Salad
Porchetta
Crab Cakes
Skirt Steak with Chimichurri Sauce
Chicken Piccata with Spaghetti
Turkey Ragout
Rich Mushroom Risotto
Sesame-Crusted Tuna Steak
Pernil
Hamachi Tacos
Mushroom Bread Pudding
Asian Pork Chops
Brussels Sprouts with Pistachios
Blackened Salmon Salad
Dill Asparagus
Kung Pao Pork
Classic Tuna Melt
Fish and Chips
Quinoa Bowl
BBQ Chicken Strips
BBQ Chicken Salad
Zucchini Pasta and Meatballs
Grilled Cheese and Bacon
Corn Dogs

Easy BBQ Pulled Pork
Persian Rice
Coconut Flour Tortillas
Green Rice
Cheesy Quinoa Broccoli Mac
Hushpuppies
P.F. Chang's Asian Lettuce Wraps
French Bread Pizzas 3 Ways
Poutine

· · · · · · · ·

EASY CHICKEN SOUP WITH RICE

Sometimes you just need the comfort of chicken soup. When you can't have the egg noodles or chicken stock filled with gluten, grab this recipe instead and sit back with a hot cup of tea. You'll feel better in no time.

PREP TIME: 20 minutes
COOK TIME: 45 minutes with precooked chicken and rice

2 tablespoons olive oil
4 carrots, sliced
2 celery stalks, cut into quarters
1 large onion, chopped
6 cups gluten-free chicken stock
1 whole roasted chicken, shredded
2 tablespoons fresh dill, chopped
2 cups brown rice, cooked
sea salt
freshly ground black pepper

1. Heat olive oil in a Dutch oven over medium heat. Add carrots, celery, and onion and cook for 10 minutes. Add chicken stock and cook until vegetables are tender, about 20 minutes.
2. Add chicken and dill to soup and cook for 5 minutes. Add rice and cook for 5 more minutes. Add sea salt and pepper to taste, and serve.

MAKES: 8 servings

· · · · · · · ·

SPINACH ENCHILADAS

This is one of my favorite dishes to make when I'm feeling vegetarian or having my non-meat-eating friends over for dinner. It also reheats wonderfully if you haven't scarfed it all down in one sitting. Beware that many store-bought enchilada sauces contain gluten. Find a gluten-free version or use my recipe for enchilada sauce below.

PREP TIME: 20 minutes
COOK TIME: 20 minutes

SAUCE
3 large tomatoes, quartered and seeded
1 jalapeño pepper, seeded and stemmed
1 whole white onion, quartered
2 cloves garlic
2 tablespoons olive oil
salt and pepper
¼ cup gluten-free chicken or vegetable stock

ENCHILADAS

1 tablespoon butter
2 cloves garlic, minced
½ cup green onions, chopped
1 bag spinach, washed
1 cup ricotta cheese
½ cup sour cream
2 cups shredded Monterey Jack
10 gluten-free corn tortillas

1. Preheat oven to 400 degrees.
2. To make enchilada sauce, place tomatoes, jalapeño pepper, white onion, and garlic on large baking sheet and cover with olive oil, salt, and pepper. Roast for 20 minutes, then remove from oven and allow to cool. Turn oven down to 375 degrees.
3. To make enchiladas, melt butter in a large saucepan on medium heat. Add garlic and onion and cook for 2 to 3 minutes. Stir in spinach and cook until wilted, about 3 minutes.
4. Remove spinach from heat and mix in ricotta, sour cream, and 1 cup of Monterey Jack.
5. Take cooled tomato, garlic, onion and pepper mixture and blend on liquefy until you have a very smooth-textured enchilada sauce.
6. Pour ½ cup of enchilada sauce on bottom of large casserole dish.
7. Warm tortillas two at a time in the microwave for 20 seconds, covered with damp paper towel. Fill each tortilla with spinach and cheese mixture as you remove from microwave, approximately ¼ cup filling per tortilla.
8. Roll tortillas and place seam-side down in baking dish. Pour enchilada sauce on top of tortillas, and

cover with remaining Monterey Jack. Bake for 20 minutes. Remove from heat and allow to cool before cutting into squares and serving.

MAKES: 5 servings

· · · · · · ·

TRUFFLE CHEESEBURGERS

Since I can't eat at Umami Burger because it's covered in gluten, I'm making my own dang truffle cheeseburgers at home. These are now a family favorite in my house and while I skip the bun altogether, grab a soft gluten-free bun and toast it up for the full experience.

PREP TIME: 15 minutes
COOK TIME: 8 minutes

TRUFFLE AIOLI

1 large egg
2 cloves garlic, minced
1 teaspoon Dijon mustard
½ cup extra virgin olive oil
½ teaspoon black truffle oil
2 teaspoons fresh lemon juice
¼ teaspoon sea salt

CHEESEBURGERS

1½ pounds ground beef
2 teaspoons truffle salt
4 slices Fontina cheese
4 gluten-free hamburger buns
1 bunch arugula

1. Heat grill to medium-high for at least 15 minutes.

2. While grill is heating, make truffle aioli. In blender, combine egg, garlic, and mustard, and blend until garlic is liquid and mixture is combined. Add extra virgin olive oil, truffle oil, and lemon juice, and blend again. Add sea salt to taste and transfer to small bowl. Allow to sit for 15 minutes before using.

3. To make cheeseburgers, combine ground beef with truffle salt and shape into 4 medium-size hamburger patties.

4. For burgers cooked to medium, grill patties for 3 to 4 minutes on each side. You can check for doneness by cutting into middle of patty. Medium means lots of pink. Cook longer for medium well or well done (no pink).

5. Before removing burgers from grill, add Fontina slices and allow to cook for 45 seconds, melting slightly. Toast gluten-free buns on grill for 1 to 2 minutes.

6. Build your truffle burger by placing patty on gluten-free bun and drizzling 1 to 2 teaspoons truffle aioli over burger. Top with arugula.

MAKES: 4 servings

· · · · · · ·

SUNDAY CHICKEN

I've gotten into the habit of roasting a chicken almost every weekend (hence, the name "Sunday Chicken"). You can use leftovers for enchiladas, chicken soup, or a pizza topping. It's the most useful recipe in my arsenal and easy to master.

PREP TIME: 15 minutes
COOK TIME: 1½ hours

> *3 cloves garlic, minced*
> *2 tablespoons butter, at room temperature*
> *1 (5-pound) roaster chicken*
> *3 cloves garlic, whole*
> *1 lemon, quartered*
> *3 cups gluten-free chicken stock*
> *1 onion, chopped*
> *4 carrots, quartered*
> *1 pound new potatoes, halved*

1. Preheat oven to 400 degrees.
2. Beat minced garlic into butter to completely combine.
3. Place chicken in large roasting pan with rack. Coat chicken skin, on top as well as underneath, with butter and garlic mixture. Place 3 whole garlic cloves and quartered lemon inside chicken cavity. Pour chicken stock into roasting pan and cover bottom of pan with chopped onion, carrots, and potatoes.
4. Roast chicken for approximately 1½ hours, flipping the bird over halfway through cooking time. Baste chicken periodically with chicken stock. Add water if necessary.
5. Using meat thermometer, check temperature after 1 hour. Chicken is done when internal temperature has reached 165 degrees.
6. Allow chicken to rest for 15 minutes after removing from oven before carving. Serve with roasted vegetables.

MAKES: 8 servings

· · · · · · · ·

LONDON BROIL

London broil is an all-purpose steak you can enjoy on a weeknight (or, heck, any night). The longer you marinate, the more tender the steak will be, but if you can allow it to sit for even 30 minutes, you'll have a delicious dinner.

PREP TIME: 40 minutes
COOK TIME: 6 minutes

> *1 to 2 pounds flank steak*
> *1 cup red wine*
> *1 shallot, minced*
> *2 cloves garlic, minced*
> *1 teaspoon sea salt*
> *1 teaspoon freshly ground black pepper*

1. In large bowl, cover flank steak with red wine, shallot, garlic, sea salt, and pepper. Allow it to rest for 30 minutes or up to 4 hours in refrigerator.
2. Remove steak from refrigerator if it's been marinating for an extended amount of time, and allow it to sit at room temperature for 30 minutes.
3. Heat grill on medium-high. Cook steak for 2 to 3 minutes per side for medium-rare, longer if you like less pink in the middle. Do not overcook or your steak will be tough.
4. Remove from grill and allow to rest for at least 15 minutes before slicing with the grain.

MAKES: 6 servings

. . . .

KALE, CHICKEN, AND GOAT CHEESE SALAD

So now you know what to do with all of that kale! Yes, it is another salad recipe, but this one will quickly become a family favorite. Kale salads also stand up very well the next day, so you can take leftovers for lunch.

PREP TIME: 20 minutes + 6 hours marinating time
COOK TIME: 7 minutes

CHICKEN

¼ cup olive oil
juice of ½ lemon
2 cloves garlic, minced
2 tablespoons chopped thyme
salt and pepper
2 chicken breasts
vegetable or olive oil for grill

DRESSING

½ cup extra virgin olive oil
¼ cup balsamic vinegar
1 teaspoon honey
1 teaspoon Dijon mustard
1 clove garlic, minced
salt and pepper

SALAD

1 head kale, deveined and roughly chopped
3 large carrots, shredded
1 ounce goat cheese
1 bunch green onions, chopped

1. Combine olive oil, lemon juice, garlic, thyme, and salt and pepper in small bowl. Using meat tenderizer, pound chicken breasts until between ½- and ¾-inch thick all around.

2. Place olive oil mixture along with chicken breasts in gallon ziplock bag and seal. Marinate chicken in refrigerator for 6 hours.

3. Remove chicken from refrigerator and allow to warm up while you oil and heat your grill on medium-high for 15 minutes.

4. Grill chicken for 5 to 7 minutes on each side, or until meat thermometer reads 160 degrees. Remove from grill and allow chicken to sit for 10 minutes before cutting into small pieces.

5. While chicken is resting, make dressing. In lidded jar, combine extra virgin olive oil, balsamic vinegar, honey, Dijon mustard, garlic, and salt and pepper to taste. Shake well until combined.

6. Toss kale and shredded carrots in large salad bowl. Add chicken and toss. Using your hands, break up goat cheese into small clumps and add to salad. Dress salad and toss. Add green onions and serve.

MAKES: 6 servings

· · · · · · ·

CUBAN-STYLE WHITE RICE AND BLACK BEANS

I love making these Cuban-style rice and beans at the beginning of the week, knowing I will have delicious gluten-free dinner options when I've had a long day and don't feel like cooking. Unfortunately, my kids love this so much that my "big pot" lasts

only a day or two. Consider doubling this recipe if
you have a house full of hungry people like I do.

PREP TIME: 15 minutes
COOK TIME: 1 hour

> 2 cups white rice
> 4 cups water
> ½ teaspoon salt
> 1 tablespoon olive oil
> 1 onion, chopped
> 5 cloves garlic, minced
> 3 cups cooked black beans, drained
> ½ teaspoon cayenne pepper
> 1 can diced tomatoes with liquid
> ½ teaspoon sea salt
> ½ teaspoon freshly ground black pepper
> ½ teaspoon white wine vinegar
> juice of 1 lime
> 1 tablespoon chopped cilantro (optional)

1. Combine white rice and water in medium saucepan.
   Salt well and heat to boil on high heat. Once water is
   boiling, turn heat down to low and cook for 20 to 30
   minutes, until rice is cooked through.
2. While rice is cooking, prepare beans. In large saucepan, heat olive oil, onion, and garlic on medium heat
   for 5 to 7 minutes, until fragrant. Add beans, cayenne
   pepper, tomatoes, sea salt, and pepper, and turn heat
   to lowest setting. Simmer for 15 minutes.
3. Remove beans from heat and add white wine vinegar and lime juice. Stir and serve over rice, with cilantro garnish if desired.

MAKES: 6 servings

· · · · · · ·

VEGGIE SOBA NOODLES

It can be tricky to find the gluten-free buckwheat version of soba noodles in a grocery store, so when I do, I buy in bulk. This easy and good-for-you dish is a lifesaver (and meal saver) in a pinch.

PREP TIME: 10 minutes
COOK TIME: 15 minutes

> 1 (8-ounce) package gluten-free soba noodles
> 1 tablespoon olive oil
> 1 clove garlic, minced
> 1 cup edamame
> 1 cup shredded cabbage
> 1 cup shredded carrots
> ¼ teaspoon sesame oil
> 2 teaspoons wheat-free tamari
> ½ teaspoon powdered ginger
> 2 scallions, chopped

1. Prepare soba noodles according to package directions.
2. Heat olive oil on medium-high in large skillet. Add garlic and cook for 2 to 3 minutes, until garlic is soft.
3. Add edamame, cabbage, and carrots to skillet and cook for 1 minute. Add sesame oil, wheat-free tamari, and powdered ginger, and cook for 2 to 3 more minutes. Before removing mixture from heat, add scallions.
4. Serve vegetable mixture on top of soba noodles. Add wheat-free tamari to taste.

MAKES: 4 servings

· · · · · · ·

AMY'S BEST PASTA EVER

The night my friend Amy brought a bowl full of tomatoes, garlic, and basil soaking in olive oil over to my house was a little bit life-changing. Not only is this dish a fun experiment, but the flavors are perfection. One note Amy gave me: You can never have too much Brie, but you can definitely have too much olive oil. So watch your portions carefully.

PREP TIME: 2 hours and 15 minutes
COOK TIME: 8 minutes

> 6 cloves garlic, halved
> 4 tomatoes, cored and quartered
> 2 tablespoons fresh basil, roughly chopped
> 2 cups olive oil
> ½ large wheel Brie
> 1 pound gluten-free pasta
> salt
> freshly ground black pepper

1. In large bowl, combine garlic, tomatoes, and basil. Pour olive oil over these ingredients and allow to marinate for at least 2 hours.
2. Two hours later, remove rind from Brie, and break up into smaller pieces. Add to olive oil mixture and set aside.
3. Prepare gluten-free pasta as package directs. When pasta is done, drain quickly and add hot pasta to large bowl with olive oil mixture. Stir to combine ingredients and melt Brie.

4. Add salt and pepper to taste, and serve immediately.

MAKES: 8 servings

• • • • • • • •

CHICKEN PARMESAN

While you can buy gluten-free bread crumbs, it's just as easy (and sometimes tastier) to toast up a few slices of gluten-free bread in the oven and crumble. Also, never underestimate the joy of pounding chicken breasts with a big ol' meat tenderizer. It's like stress relief before you start dinner.

PREP TIME: 15 minutes
COOK TIME: 25 minutes

1 egg
2 tablespoons milk
1 cup gluten-free bread crumbs
¼ cup grated Parmesan
1 teaspoon sea salt
½ teaspoon freshly ground black pepper
gluten-free spaghetti
2 boneless chicken breasts, flattened to ¼ to
  ⅛ inch with meat tenderizer
3 tablespoons olive oil
marinara sauce
4 ⅛-inch rounds fresh mozzarella

1. In large bowl, beat egg and milk together and set aside. In pie pan or large lipped plate, combine bread crumbs, Parmesan, sea salt, and pepper. Put water

on to boil for gluten-free spaghetti, and cook according to instructions on package.

2. Soak flattened chicken breasts in egg and milk mixture, and then dredge chicken breasts in bread crumb and Parmesan mixture, covering chicken completely.

3. Heat olive oil in large skillet and add chicken breasts. Fry for 5 minutes on each side or until crispy. Transfer chicken breasts to baking sheet.

4. Take 1 to 2 tablespoons of marinara sauce per chicken breast and spread over center of each chicken breast. Place 2 mozzarella rounds on top of each chicken breast and place in broiler. Broil chicken until mozzarella is melted and bubbly.

5. Remove chicken from broiler and serve with gluten-free spaghetti and more marinara sauce to taste.

MAKES: 4 servings

· · · · · · ·

WILTED GREENS

A simple side dish that goes with everything from steak to pasta. Choose your greens from the huge variety you can find at farmers' markets or in the produce section. While kale is always a good choice, branch out with Swiss chard, spinach, or collard greens.

PREP TIME: 10 minutes
COOK TIME: 10 minutes

1 bunch greens of your choice
2 tablespoons olive oil

> *1 shallot, diced*
> *2 cloves garlic, minced*
> *juice of 1 lemon*
> *salt and pepper*

1. Wash, devein, destem, and roughly chop your greens.
2. In medium skillet, heat olive oil on medium-high and add shallot and garlic. Cook for 5 to 7 minutes, until shallot and garlic have softened and slightly browned.
3. Add greens to skillet and turn heat down to medium. Constantly stirring, cook greens for 2 minutes, then remove from heat.
4. Transfer greens to serving dish, evenly distribute lemon juice over greens, and add salt and pepper to taste.

MAKES: 4 servings

· · · · · · ·

POLENTA TORTA

This epic dish will look beautiful on your table as a holiday centerpiece or at any other time of year. Again, make sure your polenta is gluten-free, and dig in.

PREP TIME: 3 hours
COOK TIME: 45 minutes

> **PESTO LAYER**
> *I like to use premade pesto as a cheat, but if you're making your own, here are the ingredients:*

½ cup pistachios, shelled

5 cloves garlic

3 cups basil, roughly chopped

½ teaspoon sea salt

1 teaspoon black peppercorns

1 cup olive oil

¼ cup Parmesan, grated

POLENTA LAYER

butter, for greasing pan

4½ cups (36 ounces) precooked gluten-free
   polenta

2 tablespoons butter

3 cups gluten-free chicken or vegetable stock

¼ cup mozzarella, grated

¼ cup Parmesan, grated

¼ cup Gruyère, grated

salt and pepper

TOMATO LAYER

3 tablespoons extra virgin olive oil

2 large or 4 small shallots, minced

2 cloves garlic, minced

2 (15-ounce) cans diced tomatoes

¼ to ½ teaspoon crushed red pepper flakes

kosher salt and freshly ground black pepper

1. Butter 9-inch springform pan. Line bottom and sides with parchment paper.

2. Prepare pesto if you have not purchased it by grinding pistachios, garlic, basil, sea salt, and peppercorns in mortar and pestle or food processor. Transfer mixture to small bowl and add olive oil and Parmesan and mix well. Set aside.

3. Heat polenta on medium in large skillet in butter and chicken or vegetable stock. After polenta is thoroughly combined with wet ingredients, add cheeses, stirring after each addition. Add salt and pepper to taste. Mix thoroughly and allow to cook for 2 or 3 more minutes on medium-low heat.

4. Remove polenta mixture from heat and spread evenly in parchment-covered springform pan. Transfer to refrigerator and allow to chill for at least 20 minutes.

5. While polenta is cooling, make tomato layer: Heat olive oil on medium in a large skillet. Add shallots and cook until soft, approximately 3 minutes. Add garlic and cook for 1 or 2 minutes. Turn heat down to low and stir in tomatoes. Add red pepper flakes and allow tomato mixture to simmer for 20 minutes. Season with salt and pepper immediately before removing from heat.

6. Remove polenta from refrigerator and spread pesto mixture evenly on top. Spoon tomato mixture on top and transfer back to refrigerator. Allow to chill for at least 2 hours before serving.

7. Remove polenta torta from springform and slice to serve.

MAKES: 15 servings

• • • • • • • •

CHEESY CAULIFLOWER PIZZA

I'll admit I had to test this pizza crust at least five times before finding the right mix and the right cooking time. The key to success with a cauliflower pizza crust is twofold: Squeeze as much liquid out as possible, and do not overcook. Once you've got it down, you may never go back to a regular gluten-free crust.

PREP TIME: 30 minutes
COOK TIME: 25 minutes

1 head cauliflower
1 teaspoon fresh basil, chopped
1 clove garlic, minced
¼ cup mozzarella, shredded
¼ cup Parmesan, grated
1 teaspoon salt
1 teaspoon fresh black pepper

TOPPINGS

½ cup tomato sauce
1 teaspoon oregano
¼ cup mozzarella, shredded
pepperoni

1. Preheat oven to 450 degrees.
2. Place cauliflower in food processor or blender and pulse until cauliflower appears rice-like. Transfer cauliflower to microwave-safe bowl.
3. Place cauliflower in microwave for 8 minutes. Remove and allow it to cool to the touch.
4. While cauliflower is cooling, combine basil, garlic, cheeses, salt, and pepper in large bowl. Set aside.
5. Place cooled cauliflower on clean dish towel and wrap towel around so no cauliflower can escape. Squeeze any excess liquid out of cauliflower. Transfer drained cauliflower into bowl with cheese mixture and combine.
6. Spray a pizza pan or baking sheet with olive oil and

arrange cauliflower mixture into 9-inch round. Spray olive oil over top of crust and bake for 10 minutes or until edges are crispy and crust is brown.

7. Remove pizza crust from oven and cover with tomato sauce, sprinkle with oregano, and add mozzarella and pepperoni to your liking. Bake for another 5 minutes or until cheese is melted and bubbly. Allow to rest for 5 to 10 minutes and serve.

MAKES: 8 servings

· · · · · · ·

BBQ SPARE RIBS

Don't be intimidated by spare ribs just because they're not on regular rotation in your house. If you wrap those ribs up in this delicious BBQ sauce (and be generous in your brushing) and cook long enough, the meat will fall off the bone. Don't forget, if you're using BBQ sauce from a jar, check for any gluten ingredients.

PREP TIME: 10 minutes
COOK TIME: 15 minutes + 3 hours

BBQ SAUCE

4 strips bacon
1 clove garlic, minced
4 cups ketchup
1 cup water
¾ cup brown sugar
1 teaspoon sea salt
½ cup apple cider vinegar
1½ tablespoons hot sauce

1½ teaspoons chili powder
¼ teaspoon ground cloves

3 pounds beef short ribs

1. Preheat oven to 250 degrees.
2. Fry bacon in large, deep skillet. Remove bacon and drain almost all bacon grease, reserving 1 teaspoon for cooking.
3. Add garlic to grease in skillet and cook for 1 to 2 minutes, until it starts to become transparent. Add ketchup, water, sugar, salt, vinegar, hot sauce, chili powder, and cloves and turn heat up to high. Bring to a boil and allow to cook for 3 to 4 minutes.
4. While sauce is cooking, crumble bacon. Add to sauce when it's off the heat. Reserve 1 cup of sauce for serving in a separate bowl.
5. Line baking sheet with aluminum foil. Place layer of BBQ sauce on foil before laying down short ribs. Brush BBQ sauce on ribs thickly, covering completely. Bake ribs for 3 hours. Remove from heat and serve immediately.

MAKES: 6 servings

· · · · · · ·

PAN-SEARED HALIBUT

I've always been afraid of cooking fish, but halibut is an easy way to go, even for the uninitiated. I always buy a fillet so I don't have to do any deboning myself, thus ensuring quick and easy meal prep.

PREP TIME: 5 minutes
COOK TIME: 10 minutes

1 tablespoon olive oil

1 clove garlic, minced

2 teaspoons coarse sea salt

2 teaspoons freshly ground black pepper

2 teaspoons thyme, minced

4 (6-ounce) skinless halibut fillets

1 tablespoon melted butter, if desired

¼ teaspoon red pepper flakes

1. Over medium heat, heat olive oil and garlic in large skillet for 2 to 3 minutes, until garlic begins to soften.
2. Combine sea salt, pepper, and thyme in medium bowl. Dredge halibut filets in mixture, covering all sides.
3. Transfer fillets to skillet and cook for 4 minutes on each side, or until slightly browned on each side.
4. Remove halibut from heat and, if desired, pour melted butter evenly over fish. Sprinkle red pepper flakes over halibut and serve immediately with Wilted Greens or with Polenta Crostini with White Beans and Kale as a side.

MAKES: 4 servings

· · · · · · · ·

SPAGHETTI SQUASH WITH PESTO

I grew up eating spaghetti squash, since it grew like wild in our garden. While we would go sweet by adding butter and cinnamon, I also like to use it as a pasta replacement. Every now and then, even my kids will eat it.

PREP TIME: 15 minutes
COOK TIME: 50 minutes

1 large spaghetti squash
3 tablespoons olive oil
salt and pepper

PESTO (OR USE PREMADE)

½ cup pistachios, shelled
5 cloves garlic
3 cups basil, roughly chopped
½ teaspoon sea salt
1 teaspoon black peppercorns
1 cup olive oil
¼ cup Parmesan, grated

1. Preheat oven to 375 degrees.
2. Cut spaghetti squash in half lengthwise, and scoop out all the seeds and strings in the center.
3. Place each half in large baking dish and drizzle olive oil over both sides evenly. Add salt and pepper to taste. Bake for 45 to 50 minutes or until fork can go in spaghetti squash flesh easily.
4. While squash is baking, prepare pesto (if not using premade) by combining pistachios, garlic, basil, sea salt, and peppercorns in food processor or blender. Remove from blender and mix thoroughly with olive oil and Parmesan. Set aside.
5. When spaghetti squash is cooked, remove from oven, and using large fork, separate flesh from sides of skin. The squash should resemble spaghetti as you separate the strands with the fork.
6. Place spaghetti squash in large bowl and cover with pesto.

MAKES: 8 servings

········

SPICY BLACK BEAN ENCHILADAS

Here's another family favorite that I make on the weekend in hopes that it will make for an easy dinner during the week. Yet again, the popularity of this dish means it's gone in two (and sometimes one!) sittings. Remember, many brands of enchilada sauce have gluten, which is why I make my own. If you're lucky enough to come across gluten-free enchilada sauce, stock up to make this dish even easier.

PREP TIME: 20 minutes
COOK TIME: 1 hour

SAUCE

3 large tomatoes, quartered and seeded
1 jalapeño pepper, seeded and stemmed
1 whole white onion, quartered
2 cloves garlic
2 tablespoons olive oil
salt and pepper
¼ cup gluten-free chicken or vegetable stock

FILLING

1 tablespoon olive oil
1 clove garlic, minced
2 (15-ounce) cans black beans, drained
¼ teaspoon cilantro, minced (optional)
½ teaspoon hot sauce
salt and pepper

TOPPING

8 gluten-free corn tortillas
2 cups Monterey Jack–cheddar mix, grated

1. Preheat oven to 400 degrees.
2. To make enchilada sauce, place tomatoes, jalapeño pepper, white onion, and garlic on large baking sheet and cover with olive oil, salt, and pepper. Roast for 20 minutes, then remove from oven and allow to cool. Turn oven down to 350 degrees.
3. While your vegetables are cooling, make your beans for the filling. Heat olive oil in a medium saucepan on medium-high. Add garlic and cook until soft, about 5 to 7 minutes. Add beans, cilantro (if using), hot sauce, salt, and pepper, and cook on medium for 10 minutes to allow all the flavors to mix. Remove from heat and allow to cool.
4. Transfer cooled vegetables to blender or food processor, add chicken or vegetable stock, and liquefy. If mixture is dry, add olive oil ¼ teaspoon at a time until texture resembles sauce, but I prefer the sauce a little thicker than store-bought. Place thin layer of enchilada sauce on bottom of 13-by-9-inch baking pan. Reserve remaining sauce for topping.
5. Heat tortillas for 20 seconds in microwave, two at a time, covered with damp paper towel. Remove from microwave and begin to assemble enchiladas.
6. Working quickly, fill one tortilla at a time with 2 to 3 tablespoons of beans. Roll tortillas and place in baking pan, seam-side down. Repeat, moving filled tortillas close to one another.

7. Cover tortillas with remaining enchilada sauce, then cover with grated cheese. Bake for 20 minutes.

   MAKES: 8 servings

· · · · · · · ·

LENTIL AND LOX SALAD

I discovered this salad in Paris at a museum restaurant. I was feeling desperate for something delicious and gluten-free in the land of baguettes, and this salad more than fit the bill. I re-created it when I came home, and it's almost as good as sitting in front of a Monet. Almost.

PREP TIME: 8 minutes
COOK TIME: 25 minutes

> 1 cup dried lentils
> 2 cups water
> salt, to taste
> 6 ounces lox
> juice of ½ lemon
> ¼ cup extra virgin olive oil
> 2 teaspoons fresh dill, chopped

1. Rinse dry lentils in a strainer with water, sorting for any debris. In medium saucepan, combine water and lentils and cook on medium-high. Add dash or two of salt. After 5 minutes, lower heat to medium and cook lentils for 20 minutes.
2. While lentils are cooking, cut lox into small pieces with sharp knife.

3. Strain cooked lentils of all water and transfer lentils to medium bowl. Salt lightly.
4. Add lox, lemon juice, olive oil, and dill to lentils and stir.

MAKES: 4 servings

• • • • • • •

BACON-WRAPPED SCALLOPS

An easy and delicious meal, you just need to make sure your grill is clean and your scallops are fresh to ensure success. Always buy sea scallops rather than bay scallops, as they are larger and easier to wrap bacon around.

PREP TIME: 10 minutes
COOK TIME: 7 minutes

> 5 to 7 slices bacon
> 1 pound large sea scallops
> 4 tablespoons butter
> ¼ teaspoon cayenne pepper
> ¼ teaspoon paprika
> dash of salt

1. Slice bacon into 4- to 6-inch pieces that fit perfectly around your scallops. Test one, then use it as a guide for the rest.
2. Using long toothpicks, wrap bacon around each scallop. Place scallops on a tray.
3. Melt butter and mix well with cayenne, paprika, and salt. Pour mixture evenly over scallops.
4. Oil grill and preheat on medium. Transfer scallops

to grill and cook until scallops are cooked through and bacon is cooked, approximately 7 minutes. Flip midway through cooking. Do not overcook.

MAKES: 4 servings

· · · · · · · ·

SMASHED POTATOES WITH BACON

Smashed potatoes are one of my most favorite things to eat and make. Which is why I try variations on the theme. Of course, one of those variations is going to be bacon. Of course.

PREP TIME: 10 minutes
COOK TIME: 1 hour

> 15 new potatoes
> 2 tablespoons olive oil
> salt and pepper
> black truffle oil
> parsley, chives, or other herb, chopped
> (optional)
> 6 slices bacon

1. Preheat oven to 450 degrees.
2. Bring large pot of water and sprinkle of salt to boil. Make sure there is enough water to cover potatoes. Boil potatoes until you can slide a fork in with little resistance, approximately 15 to 20 minutes.
3. Drain potatoes and place them, evenly spaced, on baking sheet covered in foil. Allow to cool for a few minutes, then take a clean dishtowel and press on each potato to smash, while keeping potato still intact.

4. Drizzle olive oil evenly over potatoes. Add salt and pepper, and small amount of black truffle oil to potatoes. Throw some chopped parsley, chives, or herb of your choice atop if you like. Bake for 25 to 30 minutes or until crispy.

5. While potatoes are baking, cook bacon until crispy. Allow bacon to cool, and crumble into bits. When potatoes come out of oven, sprinkle bacon bits evenly over each potato.

6. Use spatula to remove potatoes and serve with sour cream, or on their own.

MAKES: 15 servings

. . . .

STEAK AND SPINACH SALAD

A fantastic salad that you can make ahead and enjoy for lunch. I'm a big fan of the steak and spinach combo. Keep the dressing on the side until the last minute for optimal freshness.

PREP TIME: 20 minutes
COOK TIME: 10 to 14 minutes

1 tablespoon wheat-free tamari
1 tablespoon red wine
1 clove garlic, minced
½ teaspoon salt
½ teaspoon black pepper
1 New York strip steak

DRESSING

1 cup extra virgin olive oil
½ cup balsamic vinegar
1 teaspoon Dijon mustard
⅛ teaspoon coarse sea salt
½ teaspoon freshly ground black pepper

1 bunch spinach
½ cup pomegranate seeds
½ cup white mushrooms, sliced
¼ cup walnuts

1. In medium bowl, combine wheat-free tamari, red wine, garlic, salt, and pepper. Marinate steak in mixture for at least 20 minutes at room temperature.

2. Heat your grill on medium-high for at least 15 minutes. Cook steak 5 to 7 minutes on each side, depending on thickness. Check middle of steak for pinkness with knife after 5 minutes. Medium should have lots of pink left, but no red. Remove steak from grill and allow to sit for 10 minutes before slicing steak with the grain.

3. Prepare dressing by combining olive oil, balsamic vinegar, mustard, sea salt, and pepper in lidded jar and shaking to combine.

4. Assemble salad in large salad bowl: spinach, pomegranate seeds, mushrooms, walnuts, and steak on top. Dress salad and serve.

MAKES: 4 servings

. . . .

TWICE-BAKED POTATOES

I pull this old favorite out whenever I want to impress anyone who didn't grow up in Texas or Oklahoma. While this may be second nature to those of us from a certain part of the United States, it comes off as positively magical for those who have not been blessed with twice-baked potatoes as a dinner table staple.

PREP TIME: 15 minutes
COOK TIME: 1½ hours

4 large russet potatoes
½ cup milk or cream
3 tablespoons unsalted butter
salt and pepper
1 cup grated cheese of your choice

1. Preheat oven to 400 degrees.
2. Wash potatoes, poke holes in skin with fork, and wrap up with aluminum foil. Bake for 45 minutes or until there is give when you touch the skin, but they are not totally soft.
3. Remove potatoes from oven and unwrap from foil. Turn oven down to 350 degrees.
4. Using sharp knife, cut oval on top of potato and remove that area of potato skin. Using knife and spoon, carefully cut and scoop out potato and place in medium saucepan. Take care to leave body of potato intact, and upright.
5. Over medium heat, add milk or cream and butter to potato. Using potato masher, mash until smooth. Add salt and pepper to taste.

6. Place potatoes on baking sheet and assemble by spooning mashed potatoes into skins. Mashed potatoes should be coming out the top of potato skins. Divide grated cheese evenly and create cheese mound on top of each potato.

7. Place stuffed potatoes back in oven and cook for 10 minutes. Remove from oven and serve.

MAKES: 4 servings

· · · · · · ·

PARMESAN POPOVERS

All popovers are delicious, but add a little bit of Parmesan and your popovers will wow even the biggest gluten fan. Be sure you make this side dish last so that the popovers are warm and still standing when you serve dinner.

PREP TIME: 7 minutes
COOK TIME: 30 minutes

> 2 tablespoons butter, melted
> 1 cup all-purpose gluten-free flour
> 1 teaspoon sugar
> ½ teaspoon salt
> 2 eggs, room temperature
> ½ cup grated Parmesan, divided

1. Preheat oven to 425 degrees.
2. Butter 12-cup muffin or popover pan thoroughly and place it in oven to preheat for 10 minutes.
3. Combine flour, sugar, salt, eggs, and ¼ cup Parmesan with a whisk. Divide batter into 12 equal portions.

4. Bake for 10 minutes and pull pan out to sprinkle remaining Parmesan on top. Bake for 20 more minutes.

5. Remove from oven and serve immediately.

MAKES: 12 servings

. . . .

SPICY TOFU STIR-FRY

This is one of my favorite dishes, even though I'm a big fan of meat. The flavors work perfectly together, and the crunch of the crispy tofu makes for an absolutely delightful meal.

PREP TIME: 15 minutes
COOK TIME: 7 minutes

> 2 tablespoons vegetable oil
> 1 clove garlic, minced
> 1 block firm tofu, cubed
> small head cabbage, shredded
> 1 cup snow peas
> 1 cup bok choy, chopped
> 1 cup carrots, shredded
> ½ teaspoon sugar
> 3 tablespoons wheat-free tamari
> ¼ cup chopped green onions
> 2 teaspoons sesame seeds
> 1 tablespoon sesame oil
> 1 teaspoon red pepper flakes
> 2 cups cooked rice (optional)

1. Heat vegetable oil in large skillet on medium-high, add garlic, and turn down to medium.

2. Add tofu, cabbage, snow peas, bok choy, carrots, sugar, and wheat-free tamari to skillet. Moving constantly, cook for 3 to 5 minutes.

3. Add green onions, sesame seeds, sesame oil, and red pepper flakes, and cook for 1 minute more. Remove from heat and serve alone or with rice.

MAKES: 8 servings

· · · · · · ·

CHICKEN MASALA-ISH

When I complained about the lack of Indian food in my gluten-free life, a friend sent me this recipe. Knowing my love for potatoes, she thought it would make me deliriously happy. It did.

PREP TIME: 30 minutes
COOK TIME: 2½ hours

3 tablespoons butter (or ghee)
3 pounds boneless chicken thighs
salt and pepper
1 white onion, finely chopped
4 cloves garlic, minced
2 tablespoons peeled ginger, grated
2 tablespoons tomato paste
2 teaspoons chana masala
2 teaspoons ground cumin
2 teaspoons ground turmeric
1½ teaspoons ground coriander
¾ teaspoon cayenne pepper
¾ teaspoon ground cardamom
8 cups gluten-free chicken broth

> ¾ cup canned tomato sauce
>
> ½ cup heavy cream
>
> 1 pound small Yukon Gold potatoes, sliced
>   ¼ inch thick, or fingerling potatoes
>
> 2 cups cooked rice

1. Heat butter or ghee in large Dutch oven over medium heat. Season chicken with salt and pepper. Working in batches, cook chicken, skin side down, until brown, about 8 minutes. Transfer to a plate.

2. Add onion, garlic, and ginger to pot and cook until onions are soft, about 8 minutes.

3. Add tomato paste, masala, cumin, turmeric, coriander, cayenne, and cardamom, and mix until fully blended. Cook until tomato paste is beginning to darken, about 4 minutes.

4. Put chicken back into pot, and add broth, tomato sauce, and cream. Season with more salt and pepper and bring to boil. Reduce heat and simmer, partially covered, until chicken is falling apart and liquid is slightly thickened, 1½ to 2 hours.

5. Add potatoes to pot and cook until tender and liquid is thick enough to coat a spoon, about 40 minutes. While stew is cooking, prepare rice according to package directions.

6. Remove stew from heat and serve over rice.

MAKES: 12 servings

• • • • • • •

SMOKY-SWEET POTATO SOUP

You can make this simple recipe vegan by using gluten-free vegetable stock instead of gluten-free chicken broth, and you can make it full-fat and creamy by using half-and-half instead of almond milk. This balance works perfectly for me (and it's also Paleo!).

PREP TIME: 15 minutes
COOK TIME: 1 hour

1 large baked sweet potato
¼ cup almond milk
¼ cup gluten-free chicken broth
1 chipotle pepper, sliced and in
   sauce
salt
freshly ground black pepper
1 avocado, cubed

1. Preheat oven to 400 degrees.
2. Bake sweet potato for 45 minutes to 1 hour, until it's no longer firm to the touch. Remove from oven and carefully remove skin. Place skinned potato in blender or food processor.
3. Add almond milk, chicken broth, and chipotle pepper, and blend to liquefy. Add more chicken broth if you wish to have a thinner soup. Add salt and pepper to taste.
4. Pour soup into two bowls if it's still warm from baking; otherwise, heat up on stovetop or in microwave

to desired temperature. Serve immediately with avocado garnish.

MAKES: 2 servings

. . . .

CHICKEN MOLE WITH RICE

My husband has asked that I increase the frequency of chicken mole at our dinner table, but I find that I eat more of the chocolate than I cook with when I whip this up. So maybe I *should* make it more often. Yummmmm.

PREP TIME: 15 minutes
COOK TIME: 1 hour

> 1 tablespoon olive oil
> 4 pounds chicken thighs
> 1 white onion, diced
> 2 cloves garlic, minced
> 1 (14-ounce) can diced tomatoes
> ½ teaspoon sea salt
> ¼ teaspoon freshly ground black pepper
> ½ teaspoon sweet paprika
> ¼ teaspoon cayenne pepper
> ½ teaspoon cinnamon
> 1 bay leaf
> 3 ounces Mexican chocolate, roughly chopped
> 2 teaspoons brown sugar
> 6 cups white rice, cooked
> 1 tablespoon pepitas, toasted

1. In large Dutch oven, heat olive oil on high for 5 to 7 minutes. Add chicken thighs, turn heat down to

medium, and cook, while turning, for 10 to 15 minutes or until brown on all sides. Remove chicken from Dutch oven and set aside.

2. Cook onion and garlic in Dutch oven until onion is translucent, approximately 8 minutes. Add diced tomatoes and continue to cook on medium.

3. Add sea salt, pepper, paprika, cayenne, cinnamon, and bay leaf to Dutch oven and cook for 1 minute. Stir in chocolate and brown sugar, and cook until chocolate is melted and ingredients are well combined.

4. Return chicken to Dutch oven, and if liquid is needed, add ¼ cup water. Turn heat to medium-low and cook chicken in sauce for 25 minutes.

5. While chicken is cooking, prepare rice according to package directions.

6. Serve chicken on top of white rice, with toasted pepitas as garnish.

MAKES: 6 servings

· · · · · · · ·

SPICY MEATLOAF

As you can see from other recipes, we've become quite addicted to chipotle peppers and the spicy sauce they come in when you buy them in a can. I've been adding them to many dishes, but this meatloaf really benefits from the jolt of flavor. Honestly, I add a little bit more than 2 teaspoons to this recipe, but they make it incredibly spicy, so I feel more comfortable advising you all to take it easy. If you're a big fan of hot and spicy, however, feel free to experiment with your measures.

PREP TIME: 20 minutes
COOK TIME: 1 hour

1 pound ground beef
1 pound ground pork
1 egg
1 clove garlic, minced
¼ cup ketchup
¼ cup gluten-free bread crumbs
1 teaspoon sea salt
1 teaspoon black pepper
2 teaspoons chipotle pepper sauce
2 tablespoons tomato paste

1. Preheat oven to 350 degrees. Spray loaf pan with gluten-free cooking spray.
2. Combine beef and pork in large mixing bowl, using hands if necessary.
3. In small bowl, beat egg well. Add garlic, ketchup, bread crumbs, sea salt, pepper, and chipotle pepper sauce.
4. Add ketchup mixture to pork and beef, and mix completely. Again, use your hands if necessary.
5. Transfer mixture into loaf pan and shape to fit. Spread tomato paste on top and place in oven.
6. Bake meatloaf for 1 hour. Remove from oven, slice, and serve.

MAKES: 6 servings

· · · · · · · ·

CRISPY PORK LOIN

Pork loin is another family dinner staple. The most labor-intensive part of this recipe is making the marinade, which means it's pretty darn easy.

PREP TIME: 10 minutes + 2 hours marinating time
COOK TIME: 1 hour + 20 minutes standing time

> 2 pounds pork loin
> 1 cup orange juice
> 2 tablespoons sea salt
> 1 tablespoon black pepper
> 1 onion, quartered
> 3 garlic cloves

1. Score skin of pork loin and place in sealable gallon bag. Add orange juice, sea salt, pepper, onion, and garlic. Place in refrigerator for at least 2 hours and as long as overnight.
2. Preheat oven to 500 degrees.
3. Place pork, fat side up, in roasting pan in oven and allow skin to crisp for 20 minutes.
4. Turn heat down to 350 degrees and roast until pork internal temperature is 145 degrees, approximately 45 minutes to 1 hour.
5. Remove pork from oven and allow to stand for 20 minutes before slicing into medallions and serving.

MAKES: 6 servings

· · · · · · · ·

MESCLUN SALAD WITH GOAT CHEESE CROQUETTES

I'll never forget the first time I had goat cheese croquettes in a restaurant. Mind = blown. They're easy to re-create in your own kitchen and add to a simple salad. You don't want to overpower the croquettes with anything very complicated; after all, they are the star of the culinary show.

PREP TIME: 10 minutes
COOK TIME: 5 minutes

1 (3-ounce) roll goat cheese
3 tablespoons olive oil
1 egg
2 cups finely ground gluten-free bread crumbs
⅛ teaspoon salt
⅛ teaspoon pepper
1 bag mesclun greens, washed
3 medium carrots, shredded
⅛ cup slivered almonds, toasted

DRESSING

¼ cup extra virgin olive oil
juice of 1 lemon
salt and pepper

1. Slice goat cheese roll into ½-inch slices. If slices don't stay together, roll into balls and flatten between your hands. Heat olive oil over medium heat for 5 to 7 minutes. While oil is heating, prepare goat cheese.
2. Beat egg in medium bowl. Combine bread crumbs,

salt, and pepper in another medium bowl. First cover each goat cheese slice with egg, then transfer egg-covered goat cheese slices to bowl with bread crumbs and evenly cover.

3. Cook coated goat cheese slices in olive oil for 2 to 3 minutes per side to get crispy outer shell without melting cheese completely. Set aside cooked goat cheese medallions on paper towel–covered plate.

4. While goat cheese is cooking, assemble salad. Toss mesclun greens, carrots, and toasted almonds in large bowl.

5. Combine olive oil, lemon juice, and salt and pepper to taste for dressing. Shake well until completely mixed.

6. Dress salad and toss again. Layer goat cheese cro-quettes atop greens and serve.

MAKES: 4 servings

· · · · · · ·

SWEET AND SOUR CHICKEN

Re-creating our favorite dishes from Chinese restau-rants has become my part-time job in my house. Sweet and sour chicken is one of those you really can't find gluten-free in a restaurant, so naturally I created my own. You can use orange juice if you want it a little bit sweeter, but I went with pineapple as I prefer the sour over the sweet. The sriracha re-ally makes all the difference at the end of the recipe, so don't skip it!

PREP TIME: 20 minutes
COOK TIME: 35 minutes

1½ cups pineapple juice
½ cup rice wine vinegar
1 cup water
¼ cup cornstarch + 2 cups for dredging
1 egg
¼ teaspoon salt
¼ teaspoon fresh black pepper
2 cups vegetable oil
4 chicken breasts, cut into cubes
2 cups chopped broccoli
1 tablespoon sriracha
6 cups cooked rice
1 bunch green onions, chopped
wheat-free tamari (optional)

1. In medium saucepan, combine pineapple juice, rice wine vinegar, and water and heat on medium. Whisk in ¼ cup cornstarch and continue whisking until fully combined. Cook on medium for 5 more minutes then set aside.

2. Beat egg in large bowl. Next to that bowl, set up bowl with 2 cups cornstarch and salt and pepper.

3. Heat vegetable oil on medium-high in large, deep skillet until top is shimmering. While oil is heating, dredge chicken pieces in egg first, then cornstarch. Place chicken pieces in skillet and cook, turning until crispy on all sides. Remove chicken from skillet and place on paper towel–lined platter.

4. Drain vegetable oil from skillet, add chopped broccoli, and cook for 1 to 2 minutes. Place chicken back into skillet. Turn heat to low and add pineapple juice mixture and sriracha. Cook entire mixture on low for 5 more minutes. Remove from heat,

serve over rice, and sprinkle green onions on top. Season with sriracha and/or wheat-free tamari if desired.

MAKES: 8 servings

. . . .

ARUGULA, CORN, AND RED ONION SALAD

I discovered this salad at the Whole Foods premade foods counter and re-created it as my favorite summer salad. Every time summer corn hits the produce section, I grab my mandolin and a red onion and go to town. It's simple and incredibly delicious.

PREP TIME: 15 minutes
COOK TIME: 3 minutes

3 ears corn
1 small red onion
1 bunch arugula, washed
2 tablespoons white wine vinegar
1 tablespoon extra virgin olive oil
¼ teaspoon salt
¼ teaspoon freshly ground black pepper

1. Fill deep stockpot with water and heat to rolling boil. Place ears of corn in boiling water and cook for 3 minutes. Remove from water and drain.
2. Allow corn to cool before cutting kernels off the cob with paring knife. Using mandolin on smallest setting, slice onion.

3. Toss arugula, corn, and onion together in large salad bowl.

4. In lidded jar, combine white wine vinegar, olive oil, salt, and pepper, and shake until completely combined. Dress salad and serve.

MAKES: 8 servings

• • • • • • •

PORCHETTA

Oh. My. Porchetta. Even after experimenting with this recipe and eating way too much of this delicious crispy pork belly, I still have to say it's a showstopper. I love to enjoy a porchetta roll straight out of the oven, but tacos the next day are just as incredible.

PREP TIME: 30 minutes + 2 to 3 days sitting time
COOK TIME: 2½ to 3 hours

1 (5-pound) pork belly, intact
5 cloves garlic, finely chopped
2 tablespoons fennel seeds, toasted
2 tablespoons rosemary, finely chopped
2 tablespoons sage, finely chopped
1 tablespoon red pepper flakes
2 tablespoons coarse sea salt + 1 extra
    tablespoon for day of cooking
zest of 1 large lemon

1. Lay pork belly out, skin side up, and score in a diagonal pattern across skin, cutting ⅛ inch deep. Flip onto other side and do the same.

2. Using mortar and pestle, grind garlic, fennel seeds, rosemary, sage, red pepper flakes, and 2 tablespoons sea salt together. Stir in lemon zest.

3. Starting on outside of pork belly, rub half of mixture into skin using your hands to get into crevices. Flip it over, and rub remaining mixture into other side.

4. Cut 5 to 7 pieces of kitchen twine in 12-inch lengths, and lay out crosswise on a cutting board the same length as the pork belly. Place pork belly flat on top of twine and get ready to roll. You want to roll pork belly up lengthwise, grabbing twine as you roll it up tightly in a long cylinder. Tie the twine tightly around pork at ½-inch intervals.

5. Transfer pork to a dish and place in refrigerator, uncovered, for 2 to 3 days.

6. After 2 to 3 days, remove pork from refrigerator and transfer to large roasting pan with rack. Allow pork to sit at room temperature for 2 hours.

7. Preheat oven to 500 degrees. Rub remaining sea salt into skin and bake pork in roasting pan for 30 minutes. Then turn heat down to 300 degrees and roast for 1½ to 2 hours, or until internal temperature reaches 150 degrees. If skin is in need of more crackling, turn heat back up to 500 degrees and cook for 10 to 15 minutes or until skin is done.

8. Remove from heat and allow pork to stand for 15 minutes before removing twine and slicing into ½-inch rounds. Serve alone, in a tortilla with all the accouterments, or in a sandwich with gluten-free bread.

MAKES: 12 servings

. . . .

CRAB CAKES

Another really simple dish that you'll never (or very rarely) find gluten-free in a restaurant, crab cakes can be made full-size for dinner, or make them tiny for a delicious appetizer.

PREP TIME: 7 minutes
COOK TIME: 15 minutes

> 12 ounces crabmeat
> 1 cup GF panko bread crumbs
> 2 large eggs
> 3 tablespoons mayonnaise
> 1 tablespoon mustard
> 2 teaspoons chopped chives
> salt and pepper
> ½ cup olive oil

1. Combine crabmeat, bread crumbs, eggs, mayo, mustard, and chives and season with salt and pepper.
2. Form into two-bite-size patties and place on plate.
3. Heat olive oil in deep skillet on medium-high until a drop of water bounces. Working in batches, place patties in skillet. Add more oil if necessary between batches.
4. Allow patties to cook until golden brown on each side, approximately 4 to 5 minutes per side. Remove to paper towel–covered plate to drain.
5. Serve with tartar sauce or spicy chili sauce.

MAKES: 12 servings

· · · · · · · ·

SKIRT STEAK WITH CHIMICHURRI SAUCE

Dressing up a steak with a flavorful sauce makes a boring dinner exceptional. You can also slice up the steak, cover in chimichurri sauce, and make steak tacos. You'll notice this is not my first suggestion about making food into tacos—and it won't be my last. Tacos rule.

PREP TIME: 10 minutes
COOK TIME: 15 minutes

2 organic, grass-fed skirt steaks
3 cloves garlic
½ white onion, quartered
2 cups fresh parsley, destemmed
½ cup olive oil
2 tablespoons red wine vinegar
juice of ½ lime
red pepper flakes
salt and pepper

1. Allow steak to warm to room temperature while you're preparing chimichurri sauce.
2. Chop garlic and onion in blender or food processor. Add parsley, olive oil, red wine vinegar, and lime juice, and blend or puree again. Stir in red pepper flakes and salt to taste, and transfer to small bowl.
3. Heat grill on high for 5 minutes, then lower to medium.
4. Salt and pepper steaks on both sides. Heat each side on grill 4 to 5 minutes and remove from heat. Place

steaks on plate, covering with aluminum foil. Allow meat to rest for 7 to 10 minutes.

5. Slice steak with the grain, drizzle with chimichurri sauce, and serve.

MAKES: 4 servings

· · · · · · ·

CHICKEN PICCATA WITH SPAGHETTI

I'm not sure why capers are so good, but those little balls of salt pull this recipe together in the best possible manner. Again, get in some cathartic chicken pounding while you're making your piccata for dinner. It's good for you!

PREP TIME: 8 minutes
COOK TIME: 35 minutes

> ½ cup all-purpose gluten-free flour
> 4 tablespoons Parmesan, grated
> ½ teaspoon salt
> ¼ teaspoon freshly ground black pepper
> 2 large chicken breasts, flattened to ¼ inch
>   with meat tenderizer
> 1 package gluten-free spaghetti
> 4 tablespoons olive oil, divided
> 6 tablespoons unsalted butter, divided
> ½ cup gluten-free chicken stock
> 3 tablespoon brined capers, in liquid
> 2 tablespoons lemon juice

1. Combine flour, Parmesan, salt, and pepper on a plate. Coat chicken in flour mixture. Bring large pot

of water to boil for pasta. Cook pasta according to package directions.

2. Heat 2 tablespoons olive oil and 3 tablespoons butter in large skillet on medium-high heat. Working in batches to avoid crowding, cook chicken until brown on each side, approximately 8 to 10 minutes. Remove chicken and set aside.

3. Melt remaining butter in skillet and add remaining olive oil. Add chicken stock, capers, and lemon juice and cook on medium for 1 to 2 minutes until completely heated. Return chicken back to skillet and cover with sauce.

4. Serve over spaghetti, adding sauce from pan to taste.

MAKES: 4 servings

· · · · · · ·

TURKEY RAGOUT

A thick ragout over your favorite gluten-free pasta is perfect on those nights when your body demands comfort food. To make this recipe easier, you can buy premade Italian turkey sausage as long as it's marked gluten-free, or your butcher packaged it and can guarantee it's gluten-free.

PREP TIME: 20 minutes
COOK TIME: 40 minutes

SAUSAGE

2½ teaspoons fennel
1¼ pounds ground turkey
4 cloves garlic, crushed

3½ teaspoons paprika

1 teaspoon Italian seasoning

1 teaspoon ground cayenne pepper

½ teaspoon freshly ground black pepper

2 teaspoons kosher salt

2 tablespoons fresh Italian flat-leaf parsley,
    finely minced

2 tablespoons red wine vinegar

SAUCE

3 tablespoons olive oil

5 cloves garlic, crushed

½ cup yellow onion, finely diced

1 (8-ounce) can tomato sauce

2 (28-ounce) cans crushed tomatoes

2 tablespoons Italian seasoning

1 teaspoon kosher salt

1 large (26-ounce) jar of your favorite store-
    bought marinara sauce

1½ cups sliced crimini or baby portobello
    mushrooms

1 teaspoon ground cayenne pepper (optional,
    if you like it really spicy)

1. Toast fennel in frying pan over medium heat until fennel turns color slightly. Remove from heat.
2. In mixing bowl, add ground turkey, toasted fennel, garlic, paprika, Italian seasoning, cayenne, black pepper, and kosher salt. Using your hands, mix meat and spices until completely incorporated.
3. Add parsley and red wine vinegar to meat mixture. Mix well to incorporate.
4. In frying pan, cook turkey sausage over medium

heat until it's mostly cooked through. Using flat wooden paddle spoon, break up sausage to consistency you like.

5. In stockpot, heat olive oil over medium-high heat. Add garlic and onion. Cook until garlic and onions are fragrant, garlic starts to turn a bit brown, and onion is translucent.

6. Gently add tomato sauce over onions and garlic. Let cook for several minutes until it starts to bubble.

7. Add crushed tomatoes and stir gently to incorporate. Add Italian seasoning and kosher salt and stir again. Turn heat to medium-low and let cook until it bubbles.

8. Add marinara sauce and crimini or baby portobello mushrooms. Stir well to incorporate and simmer with lid on for 15 to 20 minutes.

9. Serve over gluten-free pasta and garnish with sprig of flat-leaf parsley and extra cayenne if desired.

MAKES: 6 servings

• • • • • • •

RICH MUSHROOM RISOTTO

Risotto is a saving grace for those of us who avoid gluten. Naturally gluten-free, it's the one dish you know you can find in an Italian restaurant while your gluten-eating friends are all slurping down their fettuccine Alfredo. You can add just about anything to a risotto to make it delicious, and using the liquid from the mushrooms to add an extra layer of flavor makes this dish particularly decadent.

PREP TIME: 10 minutes
COOK TIME: 45 minutes

> *4 cups gluten-free chicken stock*
> *½ pound dried mushrooms*
> *3 tablespoons olive oil*
> *1 onion, chopped*
> *2 cups Arborio rice*
> *⅓ cup Parmesan, grated*
> *sea salt*
> *freshly ground black pepper*

1. Heat chicken stock in saucepan on low and keep it simmering during entire process.
2. In large bowl, soak dried mushrooms in 2 cups water while cooking risotto.
3. Heat olive oil on medium-high in large Dutch oven and add onion. Cook onion until softened, approximately 7 minutes.
4. Add Arborio rice to Dutch oven and coat with oil and cooked onions. Turn heat down to medium, and cook for 1 to 2 minutes. Adding chicken stock ½ cup at a time, begin stirring rice continuously until it has soaked up all the stock. Continue to add chicken stock, stirring in ½ cup at a time until you are out of stock.
5. Drain mushrooms, reserving soaking liquid and setting mushrooms aside. Add mushroom water to rice ½ cup at a time while stirring constantly until you are out of water. If rice is still harder than al dente, continue to add water, ¼ cup at a time, until rice is al dente when you bite it.
6. Add mushrooms to rice and combine. Add Parmesan,

sea salt, and pepper to taste. Remove from heat and serve.

MAKES: 12 servings

• • • • • • •

SESAME-CRUSTED TUNA STEAK

The world's easiest seafood dinner starts with a choice piece of tuna steak. Since the tuna really is the star of the show, make sure you're purchasing it from a reputable fish store.

PREP TIME: 5 minutes
COOK TIME: 5 minutes

1 tablespoon wheat-free tamari
2 large tuna steaks
2 tablespoons sesame seeds
1 tablespoon olive oil
1 tablespoon butter

1. In medium bowl, evenly distribute wheat-free tamari over tuna steaks.
2. Place sesame seeds on flat plate, and roll edges of tuna steaks until completely covered with seeds.
3. Heat olive oil and butter in large skillet on medium-high until butter is melted. Transfer tuna steaks to skillet and cook until just seared, 2 minutes per side.
4. Allow tuna to sit for 1 to 2 minutes and serve.

MAKES: 4 servings

. . . .

PERNIL

I heard about this traditional Latin American Christmas dish years ago and just recently rediscovered the joy of having an entire succulent pork shoulder cooked and at the ready. Again, this pork does make for an excellent taco, but the first time you dine, you should simply slice and serve. It's that good.

PREP TIME: 10 minutes + 2 to 3 days
COOK TIME: 4 hours

5 pounds pork shoulder, fat on
6 cloves garlic
1 tablespoon oregano
3 tablespoons sea salt
1 tablespoon black pepper
3 tablespoons olive oil
1 tablespoon white wine vinegar

1. Using sharp paring knife, remove all but one edge of fat on top of pork shoulder, leaving it connected. Score entire pork shoulder with ⅛-inch cuts.
2. Using mortar and pestle, grind garlic, oregano, sea salt, and black pepper together. Transfer to small bowl and add olive oil and vinegar.
3. Using your hands, spread oregano mixture over entire pork shoulder, lifting fat to get on meat underneath.
4. Replace fat and wrap pork shoulder in plastic wrap. Place in large dish and store in refrigerator for 2 to 3 days.
5. Remove pork from refrigerator and preheat oven to 400 degrees for 30 minutes.

6. Place pork in large roasting pan, fat side up, and cook for 1 hour. Turn heat down to 300 degrees and cook for 3 more hours.

7. Remove from oven and allow pernil to rest for at least 20 minutes before carving. To carve, remove fat first and dice cracklings, carve pork, and place cracklings on top.

8. Serve as a main dish or in tortillas for delicious tacos.

MAKES: 12 servings

. . . .

HAMACHI TACOS

You know I just can't stop talking about tacos. Really, for the gluten-free, there is no more satisfying meal. While you may not be able to order a fried fish taco at a taco stand, try these hamachi tacos at home to fill that Jones. Again, talk to your fish store about getting sushi-grade tuna as you'll be eating this raw.

PREP TIME: 20 minutes + 5 hours
COOK TIME: 10 minutes

1¼ pounds sushi-grade hamachi
juice of 3 limes + 1 lime
juice of 2 lemons
½ teaspoon sea salt
1 teaspoon sriracha
½ red onion, diced
4 tablespoons cilantro, chopped
½ head iceberg lettuce, chopped
1 large tomato, chopped and diced

2 ripe avocados, peeled and cubed

gluten-free hard taco shells

1. Thinly slice hamachi and place in medium bowl. Cover in lime juice and lemon juice.
2. Add sea salt and sriracha and mix well. Place in refrigerator to marinate for 5 hours.
3. Cook hard taco shells according to package directions.
4. Assemble tacos with hamachi, topped with red onion, cilantro, lettuce, tomato, avocado, and another spritz of lime juice from a fresh lime.

MAKES: 4 servings

• • • • • • •

MUSHROOM BREAD PUDDING

I adore a sweet bread pudding, but there's something to be said about a rich, savory bread pudding to complement a special-occasion dinner. If you can find a gluten-free brioche, go for it and use the whole loaf. Otherwise, any gluten-free white bread will do for this delicious side dish.

PREP TIME: 20 minutes
COOK TIME: 1½ hours

10 to 12 slices gluten-free white bread

1 clove garlic, minced

1 teaspoon fresh thyme

¼ cup olive oil

4 tablespoons butter

1 onion, chopped

3 cups mushrooms of your choice, sliced
2 tablespoons parsley, roughly chopped
6 eggs
2½ cups half-and-half
¼ cup Fontina, shredded
coarse sea salt
freshly ground black pepper

1. Preheat oven to 375 degrees.
2. Cut bread into cubes and place in large bowl. Mix garlic, thyme, and olive oil into bread, thoroughly covering bread with oil.
3. Transfer mixture onto greased baking sheet and bake for 20 minutes.
4. While bread is baking, melt butter in medium skillet on medium-high. Add onion and cook for 3 to 5 minutes or until onion begins to soften. Add mushrooms and sauté for 10 minutes.
5. Remove bread from oven and turn temperature down to 350 degrees. Transfer bread mixture back into large bowl, add mushroom mixture, and combine. Mix in parsley.
6. In separate bowl, mix eggs, half-and-half, Fontina, sea salt, and pepper together. Pour egg mixture into large bowl with bread-mushroom mixture and thoroughly combine.
7. Pour bread pudding into buttered medium casserole dish and bake uncovered for 45 minutes.
8. Remove from oven and allow to cool and set before serving.

MAKES: 12 servings

· · · · · · ·

ASIAN PORK CHOPS

A quick, easy, and flavorful dinner that you'll go back to again and again, these pork chops are a winner whether you fry, grill, or broil.

PREP TIME: 5 minutes + 30 minutes marinating time
COOK TIME: 10 minutes

> *4 center-cut pork chops*
> *2 tablespoons wheat-free tamari*
> *1 teaspoon sesame oil*
> *1 teaspoon powdered ginger*
> *salt and freshly ground black pepper*

1. At room temperature, marinate pork chops in wheat-free tamari and sesame oil for at least ½ hour before cooking.
2. Preheat grill for 5 minutes on high, or turn on broiler.
3. Before you transfer pork chops to grill or slide into broiler, sprinkle with powdered ginger, salt, and pepper.
4. Cook pork chops 4 to 5 minutes per side. Remove from heat and allow to stand for 5 minutes before serving.

MAKES: 4 servings

·······

BRUSSELS SPROUTS WITH PISTACHIOS

This is my family's new favorite way to eat Brussels sprouts. Adding a crispy crunch makes this dish special. Yes, I did say that Brussels sprouts are "special."

PREP TIME: 5 minutes
COOK TIME: 20 minutes

> 1 pound Brussels sprouts
> 1 cup gluten-free chicken broth
> ½ cup shelled pistachios
> salt and pepper

1. Wash, destem, and quarter Brussels sprouts.
2. Heat chicken broth in large skillet on high for 3 to 4 minutes, then add Brussels sprouts and turn heat down to medium. Allow sprouts to cook for 10 minutes, or until water has been almost fully absorbed.
3. Add pistachios during last 5 minutes of cooking and turn heat up to medium-high. Salt and pepper to taste before removing from heat.

MAKES: 4 servings

·······

BLACKENED SALMON SALAD

As someone who has historically been afraid of cooking fish, salmon is another fish I've found to be surprisingly easy to prepare. Of course, if you select the freshest fish possible, it will be even better.

PREP TIME: 15 minutes
COOK TIME: 25 minutes

DRESSING

4 tablespoons freshly squeezed lemon juice
zest of 1 lemon
1 tablespoon dill, finely chopped
¼ teaspoon coarse sea salt
½ teaspoon Dijon mustard
freshly ground black pepper
6 tablespoons olive oil

SALAD

1 tablespoon ground paprika
2 teaspoons ground cayenne pepper
1 teaspoon salt
½ teaspoon ground black pepper
¼ teaspoon dried oregano
½ cup unsalted butter, melted
1 pound salmon filets, deboned
¼ cup pepitas
½ head lettuce, washed and ripped in small
  pieces

1. Prepare dressing by combining lemon juice, lemon zest, dill, sea salt, mustard, black pepper, and olive oil in lidded jar. Shake until completely combined and set aside.
2. In medium bowl, combine paprika, cayenne, salt, black pepper, and oregano.
3. Take ¼ cup of melted butter and brush both sides of salmon. Place salmon in bowl with paprika mixture and coat all sides. Drizzle one side of salmon with additional 2 tablespoons of melted butter.

4. Place salmon, butter side down, in a medium skillet, drizzle remaining butter over salmon, and cook on high heat until blackened, about 3 minutes. Turn salmon over and cook for another 3 to 5 minutes until fish is easily separated with fork. Remove from heat and separate into 2- to 3-inch pieces.

5. While salmon is cooking, roast pepitas in small pan on high heat, constantly stirring so pepitas don't burn. Roast for 2 to 5 minutes and remove from heat.

6. Assemble salad in a large bowl by placing salmon on top of lettuce, dressing the salad, and sprinkling with pepitas.

MAKES: 4 servings

· · · · · · ·

DILL ASPARAGUS

A simple, yet flavorful alternative to an old standard, this dish goes especially well with Sunday Chicken or Pan-Seared Halibut.

PREP TIME: 5 minutes
COOK TIME: 20 minutes

> 2 bunches asparagus
> 2 tablespoons olive oil
> coarse salt and freshly ground black pepper
> ¼ teaspoon red pepper flakes
> 2 teaspoons dill, chopped
> zest of 1 lemon

1. Preheat oven to 350 degrees.
2. Break ends off asparagus and place stalks on baking sheet. Cover with 1 tablespoon olive oil.

3. Bake for 10 minutes, flip asparagus over, and bake for 10 more minutes. Remove from oven and place on serving dish.

4. In lidded jar, combine salt, pepper, red pepper flakes, dill, lemon zest, and remaining olive oil. Shake until completely combined. Pour over asparagus and serve.

MAKES: 4 servings

· · · · · · · ·

KUNG PAO PORK

This is probably my favorite Chinese dish that I can no longer enjoy out at restaurants, but I actually love making it at home. Be sure to watch those chiles when you're digging in unless super hot is your go-to flavor.

PREP TIME: 35 minutes
COOK TIME: 10 minutes

6 cups cooked rice

1 tablespoon sugar

3 tablespoons water

4 tablespoons wheat-free tamari

2 tablespoons dry sherry

1 tablespoon rice wine vinegar

1½ teaspoons sesame oil

1 teaspoon + 1 tablespoon cornstarch

¼ teaspoon salt

1 pound pork tenderloin, cut into 1-inch cubes

1 tablespoon vegetable oil
8 dried whole red chiles
½ thinly sliced onion
1 teaspoon ginger, grated
½ cup unsalted dry roasted peanuts

1. Cook rice according to directions while preparing pork.
2. In medium bowl, mix sugar, water, 3 tablespoons wheat-free tamari, sherry, rice wine vinegar, sesame oil, 1 teaspoon cornstarch, and salt. Mix thoroughly.
3. Add pork to mixture. Then add 1 tablespoon cornstarch and 1 tablespoon tamari and mix until pork is covered. Cover and allow to marinate for 20 minutes.
4. Heat vegetable oil in large skillet on high heat. Add chiles and cook until chiles are blackened, approximately 1 to 2 minutes. Remove chiles and set aside.
5. Remove pork from bowl, reserving marinade, and add pork to skillet. Cook on medium-high heat, turning frequently, for 2 to 3 minutes. Add onion and ginger and cook until crispy, approximately 1 to 2 minutes.
6. Add reserving marinade and cook until it thickens and is bubbly. Add peanuts and chiles and remove from heat. Serve over rice.

MAKES: 6 servings

· · · · · · ·

CLASSIC TUNA MELT

I have a household full of people who love a good tuna melt. And I love how easy it is to make these guys happy. It's an easy lunch to pack for the kids as well.

PREP TIME: 10 minutes
COOK TIME: 10 minutes

> 1 (10-ounce) can tuna, drained
> 2 tablespoons mayonnaise
> 1 tablespoon Dijon mustard
> 4 green onions, finely chopped
> ½ teaspoon red wine vinegar
> 1 teaspoon fresh lemon juice
> salt and pepper
> butter
> 8 slices gluten-free bread
> 8 slices cheddar cheese
> 4 pickle spears

1. Combine tuna, mayo, mustard, green onions, red wine vinegar, lemon juice, and salt and pepper in medium bowl and stir well.
2. Butter 1 side of each piece of gluten-free bread and set aside on platter to assemble. Place 1 slice of cheddar on unbuttered side of each slice of bread. Divide tuna salad evenly among 4 sandwiches and close.
3. Heat small pat of butter on large skillet on medium-high and place as many sandwiches that will fit comfortably in skillet. Turn skillet down to medium and

cook until bread is brown and crispy and cheese is melted. Repeat with remaining sandwiches.

4. Slice sandwiches diagonally and serve each with pickle spear.

MAKES: 4 servings

. . . .

FISH AND CHIPS

A list of my favorite recipes wouldn't be complete if I didn't have at least a few deep-fried options. And you can't really make fish and chips without the deep-fried fish, right? You can also deep-fry the "chips" if you'd like. I just thought I'd give your deep fryer a break.

PREP TIME: 25 minutes
COOK TIME: 35 minutes

CHIPS

4 large Yukon gold potatoes
1 tablespoon olive oil
3 teaspoons coarse sea salt
2 teaspoons freshly ground black pepper

FISH

1 cup cornstarch
1½ cups all-purpose gluten-free flour
2 teaspoons baking powder
1 teaspoon sea salt
1 teaspoon black pepper
1 cup milk

1 egg, beaten
vegetable oil
1½ pounds firm white fish, such as cod or
    tilapia

1. Preheat oven to 425 degrees.
2. Slice potatoes in half, then cut into spears. Place potato spears in large bowl and cover with water. Allow to sit for at least 15 minutes.
3. Spread potatoes evenly on baking sheet. Drizzle olive oil and sprinkle salt and pepper over potatoes. Bake for 20 to 25 minutes until golden brown and crispy.
4. Place cornstarch in large bowl and set aside. In another large bowl, combine flour, baking powder, salt, pepper, milk, and egg and mix well. Allow batter to sit for 10 minutes.
5. Heat vegetable oil in large skillet or deep fryer on medium-high or 335 degrees, at least 3 inches high to cover the fish. Cut fish into long strips, approximately 1 inch in diameter.
6. Dredge fish in cornstarch, then transfer to bowl with batter and completely cover fish strips.
7. Fry battered fish for 4 to 5 minutes, turning over to ensure browning on all sides. Remove from oil and drain on paper towel–covered plate.
8. Serve fries and fish strips with tartar sauce.

MAKES: 4 servings

·······

QUINOA BOWL

This dish presents a diverse way to eat healthy, keeping your favorite vegetables in rotation to make a different meal every time you cook. If quinoa isn't your thing, substitute brown rice and go to town.

PREP TIME: 15 minutes
COOK TIME: 15 minutes

2 teaspoons + 2 tablespoons olive oil
2 cups water
⅓ cup dry white wine
½ teaspoon salt
2 cups quinoa
1 bunch kale, roughly chopped
3 tablespoons fresh lemon juice
3 teaspoons finely chopped shallots
¼ teaspoon coarse sea salt
¼ teaspoon freshly ground black pepper
½ cup pomegranate seeds

1. Heat 2 teaspoons olive oil in large saucepan on medium-high heat. Add water, wine, and salt to pan and bring to boil.
2. Add quinoa to saucepan and turn heat down to low. Cover and cook for 10 minutes or until most of liquid is gone. Add kale and cook for 5 more minutes, then remove from heat.
3. In lidded jar, combine remaining olive oil, lemon juice, shallots, sea salt, and pepper, and shake until well mixed.

4. Transfer quinoa to serving bowl and stir in pomegranate seeds, then dress with lemon juice mixture.

MAKES: 8 servings

· · · · · · ·

BBQ CHICKEN STRIPS

I started making these for the kids, but the adults snatched them up as well. If you're using premade BBQ sauce, be sure to check that label!

PREP TIME: 10 minutes + 30 minutes marinating time
COOK TIME: 15 to 20 minutes

2 large chicken breasts
2 cups gluten-free BBQ sauce (see recipe on
    page 135) + 1 cup reserved for dipping
2 eggs, beaten
2 cups gluten-free bread crumbs, finely
    ground

1. Using meat tenderizer, pound chicken breasts to ½ inch thick all around. Slice chicken into strips.
2. In medium bowl, combine chicken strips and gluten-free BBQ sauce. Allow to marinate in refrigerator for 30 minutes.
3. Preheat oven to 450 degrees. Using gluten-free cooking spray, spray baking sheet so it is well greased.
4. Place beaten eggs in medium bowl next to another medium bowl containing bread crumbs.
5. Remove chicken from refrigerator and coat with eggs, followed by bread crumbs.
6. Place chicken strips, evenly spaced, on baking sheet.

Bake for 15 to 20 minutes until crispy and cooked all the way through.

7. Remove chicken strips from oven and serve with remaining BBQ sauce.

MAKES: 6 servings

. . . .

BBQ CHICKEN SALAD

My newest go-to salad for a lunch or brunch. I love how this feels like a restaurant "big salad" I can eat safely in my own home. Don't forget to check your dressing labels! Gluten can hide out in the weirdest places.

PREP TIME: 15 minutes
COOK TIME: 20 minutes

SALAD

2 ears corn
2 boneless chicken breasts
1 tablespoon butter
1 tablespoon olive oil
1 head romaine lettuce, chopped
1 avocado, cubed
1 bunch green onions, chopped
1 cup cotija cheese, crumbled
1 cup gluten-free tortilla chips, crushed

DRESSING

¼ cup gluten-free ranch dressing
¼ cup gluten-free BBQ sauce (use a premade
    brand or see my recipe on page 135)

1. Place large stockpot of water on high heat to boil. Add corn when water reaches rolling boil and cook for 2 to 3 minutes, removing immediately and draining. After corn cools, use sharp paring knife to cut kernels off, and set aside.

2. Using meat tenderizer, pound chicken breasts to ½-inch thickness all around.

3. Heat butter and olive oil in large skillet on medium-high, allowing to bubble slightly. Add chicken breasts to skillet and cook until brown on each side and cooked through, approximately 5 to 7 minutes per side. Be careful not to overcook. Remove chicken from skillet and allow to cool.

4. While chicken is cooling, assemble rest of salad in large bowl by combining romaine, corn, avocado, green onions, and cotija cheese. Chop cooled chicken, add to salad, and toss.

5. Combine ranch dressing and BBQ sauce to make the dressing. Dress salad and add tortilla chips on top to serve.

MAKES: 6 servings

• • • • • • •

ZUCCHINI PASTA AND MEATBALLS

A Paleo pleaser, this recipe looks the best if you have one of those zoodle makers that turns zucchini into the perfect spaghetti-like shape. I like to use my mandolin on the thinnest setting to get more of a lasagna/fettuccine shape with my zucchini. Either way, it's delicious.

PREP TIME: 15 minutes
COOK TIME: 35 minutes

SAUCE

2 (8-ounce) cans organic diced tomatoes
1 tablespoon organic tomato paste
2 cloves garlic, minced
salt and pepper
3 basil leaves, chopped
½ teaspoon red pepper flakes

MEATBALLS

1 pound organic, ground turkey
1 clove garlic, minced
1 teaspoon dried, or fresh diced oregano
salt and pepper
1 egg, beaten

4 large zucchini squash

1. Combine diced tomatoes, tomato paste, garlic, salt and pepper, basil, and red pepper flakes in deep pot. Using immersion blender, blend until you reach desired consistency. Put on low heat and allow to heat up while you make your meatballs.

2. Combine ground turkey, garlic, oregano, salt and pepper, and egg in a medium bowl. Mix thoroughly, using your hands if necessary. Get in there! Form meatballs and place them in tomato sauce already heating on stove.

3. Cook meatballs and sauce on medium heat, stirring 2 to 3 times for 35 minutes or until center is cooked through.

4. Put medium pot of lightly salted water on to boil. Prepare zucchini by cutting off ends and, using vegetable peeler, peeling off alternating layers of skin to make zucchini appear to have stripes.

5. Using mandolin on first setting, carefully slice zucchini into small pasta-like pieces. Toss into boiling, salted water for 1 minute, then drain and remove.
6. Serve meatballs and sauce over zucchini noodles.

MAKES: 8 servings

• • • • • • • •

GRILLED CHEESE AND BACON

Perfect. Lunch. Period.

PREP TIME: 5 minutes
COOK TIME: 15 minutes

2 slices bacon
1 tablespoon butter
2 slices gluten-free bread
2 slices American cheese

1. Cook bacon until crispy, drain on paper towel, and set aside.
2. Prepare sandwich by buttering 1 side of each slice of bread with ½ tablespoon butter. Layer cheese and bacon inside and close sandwich.
3. Wipe out skillet and begin cooking sandwich on medium heat. Flip over after 2 to 3 minutes or until bread is toasty and cheese is beginning to melt.
4. Cook for 2 to 3 minutes on the other side or until toasty. Remove from heat, slice, and serve.

MAKES: 1 serving

· · · · · · · ·

CORN DOGS

We may not be able to order lunch from "Corn Dog on a Stick" at the mall, but that doesn't stop us from re-creating the experience in our own home, with our very own deep fryer (or deep saucepan with room for frying). I found several versions of gluten-free corn dog recipes on the Internet, which just goes to show how determined we are to get our corn dog. I like to use honey in the mix to get that State Fair Taste, but you can use either sugar or honey to sweeten.

PREP TIME: 20 minutes
COOK TIME: 3 minutes each

> 1 quart vegetable oil for frying
> 8 gluten-free hot dogs (I like Applegate)
> 8 wooden skewers
> gluten-free flour for dusting
> 2 cups gluten-free corn bread mix
> 1 cup milk
> 2 large eggs
> 3 tablespoons honey
> 2 tablespoons vegetable oil

1. Preheat oil in deep fryer on high.
2. Using paper towel, dry hot dogs and set on plate or platter. Insert skewer into each center, guiding it if necessary to keep it centered in hot dog.
3. Roll hot dogs in flour until completely covered, including top and bottom. Set aside on platter.

4. Using whisk, combine corn bread mix, milk, eggs, honey, and vegetable oil until thoroughly mixed.

5. Transfer batter to tall glass and cover platter with paper towels. Set both near your deep fryer.

6. Take your first dog, dip it into batter, and swirl it around. Pull dog out and let batter drip down to make sure it's all covered. Immediately drop it into heated fryer. After cooking for 1 minute, roll hot dog over with spoon or tongs if it has not rolled over on its own. Using tongs, remove corn dog from fryer after 2 to 3 minutes, or when dark golden brown.

7. Place cooked dogs on platter to absorb oil, then serve immediately with your favorite accouterments.

MAKES: 8 corn dogs

· · · · · · ·

EASY BBQ PULLED PORK

I can't remember the first time I discovered plopping pork chops into the Crock-Pot, but I've been doing it ever since for a simple, delicious meal. You can serve this pulled pork in gluten-free hamburger buns, or just enjoy with some sides and gluten-free beer.

PREP TIME: 2 minutes
COOK TIME: 4 hours

> *4 boneless pork chops*
> *1 bottle gluten-free BBQ sauce (or see BBQ sauce recipe on page 135)*

1. Place pork chops in slow cooker and turn to medium-high. Pour BBQ sauce over pork chops and

cover. Cook for 4 hours or until pork begins to shred apart.

2. Shred pork and serve in tacos, on sandwiches, or alone.

MAKES: 8 servings

• • • • • • •

PERSIAN RICE

A fantastic rice dish to serve alongside chicken, or even on its own. We've been making this crunchy buttery version for so long it's now a go-to side dish. It's so good, that could happen in your house as well.

PREP TIME: 10 minutes
COOK TIME: 50 minutes

4 cups water
2 cups long-grain rice
4 tablespoons butter
1 yellow onion, thinly sliced with a mandolin
sea salt
freshly ground black pepper

1. Heat water in large saucepan and add rice. Bring mixture to boil, then turn down to simmer and cook rice for 10 minutes. Remove rice from heat.
2. In heavy Dutch oven, heat 2 tablespoons butter on medium-high heat until melted. Add onion in thin layer along bottom and allow to cook until softened, approximately 5 to 8 minutes.
3. Melt remaining butter. Add partially cooked rice to

Dutch oven and pour melted butter over rice. Sprinkle sea salt and pepper over rice. Cover and cook rice on low heat for 30 minutes or until crust forms along bottom and makes rice difficult to remove.

4. Remove rice from Dutch oven and serve.

MAKES: 8 servings

· · · · · · ·

COCONUT FLOUR TORTILLAS

My favorite thing about these tortillas is that you can add an extra egg white, and the texture becomes more naan-like. You can enjoy that version with Chicken Masala-ish (page 149).

PREP TIME: 10 minutes
COOK TIME: 5 minutes per tortilla

> 2 egg whites
> 1 tablespoon coconut flour
> 2 tablespoons coconut milk
> ⅛ teaspoon baking powder
> coconut oil

1. Beat egg whites until fluffy. Whisk in coconut flour, coconut milk, and baking powder. Mix well until smooth. Add more coconut milk if mixture seems thick. You want it to be thin enough that it pours out easily and spreads to pan's edges.

2. Heat coconut oil on medium heat in skillet (about 2 teaspoons per tortilla). Pour enough batter in so that it swirls around to edge of skillet. Cook for 2 to

3 minutes or until edges come up easily with spatula. Flip tortilla and cook 1 to 2 minutes longer until brown.

3. Serve with toppings of your choice.

MAKES: 2 tortillas

. . . .

GREEN RICE

One of my favorite dishes to serve with any of the Mexican dishes I make, this recipe works especially well with Spicy Black Bean Enchiladas (page 139). Note: If you have friends or family with the cilantro problem (that is, it tastes like soap to them), omit the cilantro and up your parsley.

PREP TIME: 10 minutes
COOK TIME: 45 minutes

  2½ cups gluten-free chicken broth, divided
  1 cup fresh flat-leaf parsley
  ½ cup fresh cilantro
  2 green chiles (poblano, jalapeño, or your preference), seeded and destemmed
  2 cloves garlic
  1 shallot
  3 tablespoons olive oil
  2 cups white rice

1. In food processor or blender, combine ½ cup chicken broth, parsley, cilantro, chiles, garlic, and shallot. Pulse until mixture is liquefied.

2. In large saucepan, heat olive oil on medium-high and add rice. Stir rice for 5 to 7 minutes, moving rice frequently to brown evenly.
3. Add remaining chicken broth and parsley mixture to rice, and bring to boil. Turn down heat to low, and cook for 35 to 40 minutes or until tender.
4. Remove from heat and serve with beans or other main dish.

MAKES: 6 servings

· · · · · · ·

CHEESY QUINOA BROCCOLI MAC

Once I made this for my daughter's class when we were demonstrating what could be made with a box of vegetables from the CSA our school supports. It was gone in 5 minutes flat.

PREP TIME: 15 minutes
COOK TIME: 30 minutes

> 2 cups water
> 1 cup quinoa
> ½ cup gluten-free vegetable stock
> 1 cup broccoli, chopped
> 1 cup cheddar cheese, shredded

1. Bring water to boil in medium saucepan. Add quinoa once water is at rapid boil, and turn down heat to low. Allow quinoa to cook for 20 minutes.
2. Turn heat under quinoa down to lowest setting to simmer. Immediately add vegetable stock and broccoli to saucepan and cook for 5 minutes.

3. Add cheddar cheese and combine until completely melted. Remove saucepan from heat and serve.

MAKES: 6 servings

. . . .

HUSHPUPPIES

This recipe takes me back to the time of Long John Silver's. While there's no way I could eat there today, I can at least pretend with this gluten-free version of a fun seafood side.

PREP TIME: 7 minutes
COOK TIME: 6 minutes per batch

½ cup all-purpose gluten-free flour
¼ teaspoon baking soda
½ cup gluten-free cornmeal
1 teaspoon salt
½ teaspoon freshly ground black pepper
1 egg
½ cup buttermilk
1 shallot, diced
3 cups vegetable oil

1. Combine flour, baking soda, cornmeal, salt, and pepper in medium bowl.
2. In separate bowl, beat egg and buttermilk together. Add shallot to mixture and thoroughly combine. Add to dry mixture, just combining. Do not overmix.
3. Heat oil in deep pot or cast iron skillet on medium-high. Use small amount of test batter to see if oil is hot enough to begin frying hushpuppies.

4. Using tablespoon, drop balls of hushpuppy batter into oil. Leave plenty of room in skillet, working in batches if necessary. Do not crowd hushpuppies! If hushpuppies start to burn on outside faster than cooking on inside, lower temperature to medium.

5. Cook hushpuppies until golden brown, approximately 3 minutes on each side, flipping with slotted spoon if dough does not flip itself. Remove from oil and allow to drain on paper towel. Serve hushpuppies with tartar sauce, or as a side to chili, soup, or fried fish.

MAKES: 15 servings

· · · · · · · ·

P.F. CHANG'S ASIAN LETTUCE WRAPS

I probably spend too much time at P.F. Chang's now that they have a gluten-free menu and gluten-free plates designated by markings. I still can't get enough of their lettuce wraps, though, so I re-created them at home.

PREP TIME: 20 minutes
COOK TIME: 15 minutes

1 tablespoon + 2 teaspoons sesame oil
1 pound ground chicken
2 tablespoons minced garlic
1 tablespoon wheat-free tamari
2 teaspoons fresh ginger, minced
1 small bunch green onions, sliced
1 tablespoon rice wine vinegar

3 teaspoons sriracha sauce
1 (8-ounce) can sliced water chestnuts,
    drained and finely chopped
salt
roasted peanuts, chopped
butter lettuce leaves, rinsed and drained
wheat-free tamari or spicy mustard for
    dipping (optional)

1. Heat 1 tablespoon sesame oil on medium heat in skillet. Add ground chicken and cook until browned, stirring frequently and breaking into small pieces.
2. Add garlic, wheat-free tamari, ginger, green onions, rice wine vinegar, and sriracha and cook for 1 minute. Remove from heat.
3. While mixture is still hot, add water chestnuts, another dash of sesame oil, salt, and peanuts, and mix.
4. Serve in a leaf of lettuce with dipping sauces, if desired, on the side.

MAKES: 6 servings

. . . .

FRENCH BREAD PIZZAS 3 WAYS

Again, my 1980s upbringing is showing, as I love a frozen French bread pizza. Since I buy large frozen gluten-free baguettes, I usually make several French bread pizzas and create different toppings depending on what the hungry crowd wants. Here are three winning combinations.

PREP TIME: 10 minutes
COOK TIME: 15 minutes

1 loaf gluten-free French bread
8 tablespoons marinara sauce
1 cup shredded mozzarella
¼ cup gluten-free pepperoni
¼ cup broccoli, chopped into small pieces

1. Preheat oven to 400 degrees.
2. Halve French bread and slice into four 6-inch-long pieces.
3. Cover each piece of French bread with 2 tablespoons marinara sauce. Follow with mozzarella evenly divided between slices. Add pepperoni, broccoli, or leave it alone with only cheese.
4. Bake for 10 to 15 minutes or until bread is brown and cheese is melted.

MAKES: 4 servings

· · · · · · ·

POUTINE

This delicious, rich, and insane Canadian delight is not something we gluten-free types can have outside of our own homes. So be sure you nail it when you're whipping up a batch *chez vous*. Tips: European-style butter, such as Kerrygold, has a higher fat content and thus produces a richer gravy taste. Rather than using a gravy browning and seasoning liquid, this gravy recipe calls for gluten-free liquid smoke to give the gravy more depth of flavor. A note about the flour-and-butter roux: It's normal for the roux not to clump until after you've begun adding the beef broth. Don't add more flour.

PREP TIME: 25 minutes
COOK TIME: 45 minutes

FRENCH FRIES

3 russet potatoes, washed and sliced
5 cups water
3 tablespoons kosher salt
4 cups vegetable oil

GRAVY

3 tablespoons European-style butter
4 tablespoons all-purpose gluten-free flour
3½ cups gluten-free beef broth
1½ teaspoons Wright's Hickory Liquid Smoke
1 teaspoon kosher salt
1 teaspoon poultry seasoning or Italian
    seasoning (or more to taste)
½ teaspoon white pepper

8 ounces plain cheese curds
3 tablespoons freshly chopped flat-leaf
    parsley

1. Wash and dry potatoes. Slice into French fry–size sticks.
2. In deep pot or bowl, mix water and kosher salt. Stir to dissolve salt. Submerse potatoes in salt water and soak for 1 hour.
3. Remove potatoes from water and pat dry.

4. Heat vegetable oil in deep frying pan on medium-high heat. Turn heat down to medium and add French fries and cook until golden brown.

5. Remove fries from heat and drain on paper towel–covered plate. Transfer to 250-degree oven to keep warm if necessary.

6. In saucepan over medium heat, melt butter. Whisk in flour to create a roux. Add ½ cup of beef broth at a time, continuing to whisk mixture. As broth is incorporated and begins to look like gravy, continue adding ½ cup of broth at a time and whisking until completely smooth.

7. Add liquid smoke and whisk in.

8. Whisk in kosher salt, poultry seasoning or Italian seasoning, and white pepper.

9. Reduce heat to low and allow mixture to bubble and thicken. When desired consistency is reached, remove from heat.

10. To assemble poutine, place portion of French fries in each dish. Add cheese curds to French fries and pour gravy over top of cheese curds.

11. Garnish each dish with about ½ tablespoon of parsley.

MAKES: 6 servings

•DESSERTS•

Lemon Bars
Sugar Cookie Cheesecake
Brownies with Pumpkin Bourbon Sauce
Cheesecake Ice Cream
Buckeyes
Bourbon Joe Cake

Caramel Popcorn Sundae
Deep-Fried Chocolate Cream Cookies
Chocolate Beet Bundt Cake
Lemon-Raspberry Ice
Mini Ice Cream Pecan Balls
Pumpkin Pound Cake

·······

LEMON BARS

The classic lemon bar goes gluten-free! With this much butter in the crust, no one is going to notice the difference. Win.

PREP TIME: 15 minutes
COOK TIME: 40 minutes

1 cup (2 sticks) butter, room temperature
2 cups + ¼ cup all-purpose gluten-free flour
½ cup + 1½ cups sugar
4 eggs
juice of 2 lemons
powdered sugar for dusting

1. Preheat oven to 350 degrees. Grease 9-by-13-inch pan.
2. In medium bowl, blend together butter, 2 cups flour, and ½ cup sugar. Transfer batter into greased pan and bake for 20 minutes.
3. While crust is baking, combine ¼ cup flour and 1½ cups sugar in medium bowl. In a separate bowl, beat eggs, and add in lemon juice. Pour lemon juice mixture into sugar and flour and combine completely.
4. Pour mixture over crust and bake for 20 more minutes.

5. Allow to cool for at least 30 minutes before sifting powdered sugar on top. Cut into squares and serve.

MAKES: 12 servings

· · · · · · · ·

SUGAR COOKIE CHEESECAKE

Now this is decadence. Definitely make this cheesecake when you have a crowd over, because it makes a huge amount of deliciousness. Also, you don't want that much dairy in your body at one time.

PREP TIME: 20 minutes
COOK TIME: 1 hour

CRUST

1 cup (2 sticks) butter, softened
½ cup sugar
1 large egg
1 tablespoon vanilla extract
3 cups all-purpose gluten-free flour
½ teaspoon baking powder
½ teaspoon salt

CHEESECAKE

3 (8-ounce) blocks of cream cheese, softened
3 eggs
1 tablespoon vanilla extract
1 cup sugar + ½ cup more for sprinkling

1. Preheat oven to 350 degrees. Grease a 9-inch pie or tart pan.

2. To make sugar cookie crust, beat butter and sugar with hand mixer until blended. Increase speed to high; beat until light and creamy. On low speed, beat in egg and vanilla. Beat in flour, baking powder, and salt until blended.

3. On lightly floured surface with floured rolling pin, roll dough out into a circle about ¼ inch thick. Place cookie dough into pie pan and form a crust.

4. To make cheesecake filling, combine cream cheese, eggs, vanilla, and 1 cup sugar in large bowl and beat with hand mixer on medium until thoroughly combined. Transfer to pie pan and bake for 1 hour, or until filling is firm and top is golden brown.

5. Allow cheesecake to cool, then remove from pan and place on cake stand or tray. Sprinkle entire cheesecake with approximately ½ cup sugar. Slice and serve.

MAKES: 8 servings

• • • • • • •

BROWNIES WITH PUMPKIN BOURBON SAUCE

This is absolutely one of my fall favorites. While you could roast and puree a sugar pumpkin, it's just as delicious if you pick up a can of pumpkin puree at the grocery store. And much quicker from start to getting that brownie into your mouth.

PREP TIME: 20 minutes
COOK TIME: 35 minutes

BROWNIES

2 cups sugar

1½ cups all-purpose gluten-free flour

½ teaspoon baking powder

½ teaspoon salt

½ cup cocoa powder

4 eggs

1 cup (2 sticks) butter, melted

1 teaspoon vanilla extract

SAUCE

1 packed cup brown sugar

½ cup half-and-half

4 tablespoons butter

pinch salt

1 tablespoon vanilla extract

½ cup pumpkin puree

2 tablespoons bourbon

1. Preheat oven to 350 degrees. Grease 9-by-13-inch baking pan.
2. Combine sugar, flour, baking powder, salt, and cocoa powder in large bowl.
3. In small bowl, beat eggs until fluffy. Add melted butter and vanilla.
4. Mix liquid ingredients into dry, combining completely. Pour mixture into baking pan and bake for 25 minutes, or until toothpick comes out clean from center of pan. Remove from oven and allow brownies to cool.
5. While brownies are cooling, make pumpkin sauce: Heat brown sugar, half-and-half, butter, and salt in saucepan over medium-low heat. Cook while whisk-

ing gently for 5 to 7 minutes, until mixture gets thicker. Add vanilla and cook another minute to thicken further.

6. Remove sauce from heat and mix in pumpkin puree and bourbon. Allow mixture to cool for 1 or 2 minutes, then pour over brownies. Let stand for at least 30 minutes before cutting brownies into squares and serving.

MAKES: 12 servings

· · · · · · · ·

CHEESECAKE ICE CREAM

You'll need an ice cream maker for this, and I highly recommend having one anyway, so you'll never feel at a loss for homemade dessert. The trick to making this creamy and delicious is to thoroughly whip the cream cheese so that there are no lumps.

PREP TIME: 10 minutes + 2 hours freeze time

> 12 ounces cream cheese, cut into small
>   pieces
> 14 ounces sweetened condensed milk
> 2 cups half-and-half
> 2 teaspoons vanilla extract
> 1 teaspoon lemon juice
> ½ teaspoon almond extract
> 5 to 10 gluten-free graham crackers, crushed

1. Using hand mixer, combine cream cheese and sweetened condensed milk until smooth. Do not leave any lumps.

2. Mix in half-and-half, vanilla, lemon juice, and almond extract. Place mixture in refrigerator for 2 hours.
3. Place chilled mixture in ice cream maker and follow manufacturer's instructions. Remove ice cream and serve with crushed graham crackers sprinkled on top.

MAKES: 10 servings

. . . .

BUCKEYES

You can't go wrong with this dessert from the great state of Ohio. I used to make the peanut butter balls, place them between two gluten-free pretzels, and dip them in chocolate, until a native Ohioan schooled me in the proper buckeye procedure. I would enjoy this peanut buttery treat either way.

PREP TIME: 20 minutes
COOK + FREEZE TIME: 2 hours + 10 minutes

½ cup (1 stick) unsalted butter, softened
1 cup peanut butter
1½ cups powdered sugar, sifted
½ teaspoon vanilla extract
¼ cup all-purpose gluten-free flour
12 ounces semisweet chocolate, roughly
*   chopped*
2 ounces bittersweet chocolate, roughly
*   chopped*

1. Using hand mixer, combine butter, peanut butter, powdered sugar, and vanilla, and beat until mixture is smooth. Add flour and mix completely.

2. On cookie sheets lined with parchment paper, roll mixture into 1-inch balls and place in freezer for at least 1 hour.

3. Combine both chocolates in top of a double boiler over medium heat. Stir until smooth. Remove from heat.

4. Using a skewer or a fork, dip peanut butter balls into melted chocolate, completely covering. Place on new sheet of parchment paper, and freeze for another hour.

MAKES: 50 servings

· · · · · · · ·

BOURBON JOE CAKE

You can see a theme here, and it's the amazing combo of bourbon and chocolate. I played around with the measurements for this cake until it turned out perfectly moist. It will even stand up for a few days longer than most gluten-free treats.

PREP TIME: 20 minutes
COOK TIME: 35 minutes

1¼ cups granulated sugar

¾ cup butter

½ cup unsweetened cocoa powder

2 eggs

1 teaspoon vanilla extract

1½ cups gluten-free all-purpose flour

1 teaspoon baking powder

¼ teaspoon baking soda

¾ cup milk

¼ cup bourbon

2 tablespoons instant coffee crystals

GLAZE

2½ cups sifted powdered sugar

2 tablespoons unsweetened cocoa powder

1 tablespoon bourbon

1¼ teaspoons vanilla extract

4 tablespoons brewed coffee

1. Preheat oven to 350 degrees.
2. To make cake, heat sugar, butter, and cocoa powder in large saucepan over medium heat until butter melts, stirring constantly. Remove from heat. Add eggs and vanilla; beat lightly until just combined.
3. Stir together flour, baking powder, and baking soda in bowl; set aside. In a separate bowl, stir together milk and bourbon; stir in coffee crystals. Add flour mixture and milk mixture alternately to chocolate mixture, beating by hand after each addition.
4. Pour into greased 9-by-13-inch baking pan and bake for 25 minutes or until toothpick comes out clean from center. Allow to cool for at least 30 minutes.
5. While cake is cooling, make glaze: Stir together powdered sugar, cocoa powder, bourbon, and vanilla. Add brewed coffee.
6. Pour glaze over cooled cake and allow it to cool as well. Slice and serve with vanilla ice cream.

MAKES: 16 servings

· · · · · · ·

CARAMEL POPCORN SUNDAE

I first had this popcorn sundae at Gramercy Tavern in New York City. I decided to make my own and tweak it just a little bit to make it gluten-free and easy. It looks great if you're trying to impress some fancy friends, and it offers a variety of deliciousness in each bite.

PREP TIME: 20 minutes
COOK TIME: 1 hour

3 cups popcorn, popped
¼ cup butter
½ cup (1 stick) brown sugar
2 tablespoons corn syrup
1 teaspoon vanilla extract
dash of sea salt
1 pint vanilla ice cream
whipped cream
½ cup fresh blueberries

1. Preheat oven to 250 degrees.
2. Place popped popcorn on baking sheet covered in parchment paper.
3. In medium saucepan, combine butter, brown sugar, and corn syrup, and heat to boil. Allow to cook without stirring for 3 minutes.
4. Remove mixture from heat, and add vanilla and salt. Pour mixture over popcorn and distribute evenly. Bake for 30 minutes, then remove and stir. Return to oven and bake for 15 more minutes. Remove and cool.

5. In tall glass or ice cream sundae glass, layer sundae ingredients. Using ice cream scoop, place 1 small scoop of ice cream in glass. Top with 2 tablespoons of caramel popcorn. Repeat ice cream and popcorn layer. Add whipped cream to your liking, then top with fresh blueberries.

MAKES: 4 servings

. . . .

DEEP-FRIED CHOCOLATE CREAM COOKIES

Why, yes, I *did* grow up going to the state fair—why do you ask? It's true that every now and then the urge to deep-fry something crazy just takes over me and my kitchen. Since you can find a variety of gluten-free Oreo-esque cookies, this seemed like the natural next step. If you're serving this fancy-style, feel free to drizzle chocolate syrup on top of the deep-fried cookies. But really, a dough-covered cookie is kind of enough.

PREP TIME: 10 minutes
COOK TIME: 5 minutes each + 10 minutes resting time

> 2 quarts vegetable oil for frying + 2 teaspoons additional oil
> 1 cup all-purpose gluten-free flour
> 1 teaspoon baking powder
> ¼ cup sugar
> 1 egg
> 1 cup milk

1 teaspoon vanilla extract
1 package gluten-free chocolate cream-filled
cookies

1. Using deep fryer or very deep skillet, heat 2 quarts vegetable oil on medium-high.
2. Combine flour, baking powder, sugar, egg, milk, vanilla, and 2 teaspoons vegetable oil in deep bowl and mix well until there are no lumps. Allow to sit for 10 minutes.
3. Dip cookies into batter and fully cover before putting into hot oil. Cook for 3 to 5 minutes or until batter is golden brown. Remove from oil and allow to drain on paper towel–covered plate.

MAKES: 16 servings

· · · · · · · ·

CHOCOLATE BEET BUNDT CAKE

This recipe came about when I had a CSA box full of beets and wanted to make them disappear—and quickly. At first I was skeptical (just like my kids) about a cake with vegetables, but every time I make this, I get rave reviews.

PREP TIME: 30 minutes
COOK TIME: 55 minutes

3 large beets
6 cups water
1 cup (2 sticks) butter, softened and divided
1½ cups dark brown sugar
1 teaspoon vanilla extract

3 eggs

4 ounces semisweet chocolate

2 cups all-purpose gluten-free flour

2 teaspoons baking soda

¼ teaspoon salt

powdered sugar for dusting

1. Preheat oven to 375 degrees.
2. Clean and cut beets into 2-inch chunks. Boil water, then place beets into boiling water. Allow to cook for 15 to 20 minutes, until fork can easily slide inside.
3. Remove beets from heat, drain, and allow to cool. When beets have cooled, puree in blender or food processor. Set aside.
4. Combine ¾ cup of softened butter and brown sugar, and mix well with electric mixer. Add beets, vanilla, and eggs, and mix well.
5. Melt remaining butter with chocolate, and add to mixture.
6. Combine flour, baking soda, and salt; add to creamed mixture and mix well. Pour into greased and floured Bundt cake pan and bake for 45 to 55 minutes or until toothpick in center comes out clean.
7. Allow cake to cool completely before removing from pan. Sift powdered sugar over top, slice, and serve.

MAKES: 12 servings

· · · · · · ·

LEMON-RASPBERRY ICE

It's true that this recipe can be labor intensive, but it's great in the summer. And you won't feel guilty serving this to the neighborhood kids; that is, if you don't slurp it all down first.

PREP TIME: 10 minutes
COOK TIME: 5 minutes + 4 hours freezer time

10 raspberries + 8 for garnish
2 cups sugar
1 cup water
1½ cups fresh lemon juice
8 lemon slices

1. In a blender, liquefy raspberries to make juice.
2. In deep saucepan, combine sugar and water and cook on low heat until sugar has completely dissolved.
3. Remove sugar from heat, and add lemon and raspberry juices.
4. Transfer liquid to large container, preferably metal for easier freezing. Place mixture without lid in freezer for 4 hours, stirring every 30 minutes to scrape down ice crystals.
5. Using ice cream scoop, serve with a raspberry and a lemon slice after completely frozen.

MAKES: 8 servings

. . . .

MINI ICE CREAM PECAN BALLS

You've got your ice cream, you've got your fudge, and you've got your pecans. I mean, it doesn't get much better than that. Or to quote my five-year-old, "It's like an ice cream sundae in a ball of joyness!"

PREP TIME: 15 minutes
FREEZE TIME: 45 minutes

> ½ gallon vanilla ice cream
> 2 cups chocolate fudge sauce
> 2 cups whole pecans, shelled
> whipped cream

1. Working with an ice cream scoop, form balls of slightly thawed vanilla ice cream somewhere between the size of a golf ball and a tennis ball. Place on parchment paper–covered tray and freeze for 45 minutes. (Rinse hands in lukewarm water between rolling to help keep the chill away.)
2. Remove ice cream balls from freezer and immediately transfer to small dishes.
3. Cover with chocolate sauce, arrange desired amount of pecans on balls, and top with dollop of whipped cream.

MAKES: 12 to 15 balls

· · · · · · · ·

PUMPKIN POUND CAKE

Traditional pound cakes have lots of butter, but this gluten-free pumpkin pound cake is a bit lighter because a normal amount of butter would weigh it down. The key to allowing the cake to achieve the right consistency as well as maintain moisture for several days is whipped cream cheese.

PREP TIME: 20 minutes
COOK TIME: 30 minutes

> 8 tablespoons European-style butter, at room temperature
> 4 ounces whipped cream cheese
> 1½ cups granulated cane sugar
> 3 large eggs
> 1 teaspoon vanilla extract
> 1 cup organic unsweetened pumpkin puree
> 1¾ cups all-purpose gluten-free flour
> 1½ teaspoons baking powder
> ¼ teaspoon kosher salt
> ½ teaspoon ground cinnamon
> 2 cups water (keep separate from recipe)

1. Preheat oven to 300 degrees.
2. In a stand mixer, beat softened butter and whipped cream cheese on medium-low speed until creamy and fluffy.
3. Gradually add sugar, beating until incorporated. Add eggs, one at a time, beating until yolks disappear. Add vanilla and pumpkin puree and continue

mixing until fully incorporated. It's normal for mixture to look slightly grainy or curdled.

4. In medium bowl, sift together flour, baking powder, kosher salt, and cinnamon.

5. Gradually add flour mixture to stand mixer and mix until fully incorporated. Batter will be sticky. Spray 4 mini loaf pans with coconut oil spray and spoon batter into loaf pans until halfway full. Smooth out tops with spoon or spatula.

6. In ovenproof dish, such as Pyrex glass dish, add 2 cups water. Put dish on bottom rack of oven.

7. Bake pound cake on middle rack of oven for 30 minutes or until toothpick inserted in center comes out clean. Remove from oven and cool on cooling rack.

8. Serve immediately or store in plastic ziplock bag or airtight container for up to 5 days.

MAKES: 4 small loaves

•COCKTAILS AND BEVERAGES•

Strawberry Lemonade

Pumpkin Spice Latte

Hibiscus Gimlet

Limoncello

Jalapeño Margarita

Raspberry Vodka Refresher

The Perfect G&T

Lillet Blanc Martini

· · · · · · ·

STRAWBERRY LEMONADE

I love to make lemonade in the summertime, and when strawberry season hits, this refreshing drink is just divine.

PREP TIME: 20 minutes
COOK TIME: 5 minutes + 30 minutes chill time

> 2 cups sugar, divided
> 8 cups water, divided
> 10 lemons
> 20 strawberries, destemmed
> Sliced strawberries and lemon slices for
> garnish

1. In small saucepan, mix 1½ cups sugar with 1 cup water and heat until sugar is completely dissolved. Remove from heat and allow to cool to room temperature. Then transfer to refrigerator and cool for 30 minutes.
2. Juice lemons to make 1½ cups of fresh lemon juice.
3. Combine destemmed strawberries and ½ cup sugar in blender to liquefy. Scrape down sides and transfer to bowl.
4. Combine cooled simple syrup, fresh lemon juice, and 7 cups of water in large pitcher and mix well. Add strawberry mixture and stir until completely combined. Garnish a glass with strawberry and lemon slices and serve over ice.

MAKES: 15 servings

· · · · · · ·

PUMPKIN SPICE LATTE

Once fall comes around, those of us who are gluten-free also want fancy coffee-shop drinks. The problem is, we can't always know if the flavored syrups have barley malt or not. I also make this dairy-free thanks to So Delicious Pumpkin Spice coconut milk. It's the easiest way to go here, and it's amazing.

PREP TIME: 7 minutes

2 espresso shots or 1 cup strong coffee
1 cup So Delicious Pumpkin Spice coconut milk, divided
1 teaspoon honey or other sweetener, or more to taste
1 teaspoon pure pumpkin puree
1 teaspoon vanilla extract
½ teaspoon pumpkin pie spice + more for sprinkling
nondairy whipped topping
cinnamon for sprinkling

1. Brew up espresso or strong coffee, and keep it hot.
2. In small bowl, combine ½ cup So Delicious Pumpkin Spice coconut milk, honey, pumpkin puree, vanilla, and ½ teaspoon pumpkin pie spice. Whisk until thoroughly blended. Pour coffee into large mug, and add coconut milk mixture.
3. Pour rest of coconut milk into large cup or narrow container. Using milk foamer (or a very strong arm and a whisk for a long time), beat milk until foamy. Add milk foam on top of coffee.

4. Top with nondairy topping and sprinkle with pumpkin pie spice and cinnamon.

MAKES: 1 serving

· · · · · · ·

HIBISCUS GIMLET

I was planning on re-creating P.F. Chang's Black Tea Gimlet when I came across Absolut Hibiscus Vodka in the grocery store. I tried it out instead, and I'm very happy with my tea flavor choice.

PREP TIME: 5 minutes + 30 minutes chill time for glass

> *ice*
> *2 ounces Absolut Hibiscus Vodka*
> *1 ounce St. Germain Elderflower Liqueur*
> *½ ounce fresh-squeezed lime juice*
> *lime wedge for garnish*

1. Chill large martini glass in freezer for at least 30 minutes.
2. Fill cocktail shaker with ice. Add vodka, liqueur, and lime juice. Shake until frost forms on outside of shaker, then pour into martini glass.
3. Garnish with lime wedge and serve.

MAKES: 1 serving

· · · · · · ·

LIMONCELLO

A little bit of limoncello goes a long way, so if you're making this batch, just know you'll have it hanging around the house for months. Perhaps plan a limoncello party, or buy small bottles to give as gifts during the holidays. Or hey, if you're a huge limoncello fan, keep it for yourself. No judgment.

PREP TIME: 20 minutes
COOK TIME: 5 minutes
REST + CHILL TIME: 5 days + 4 hours

> *10 lemons*
> *1 (750-milliliter) bottle vodka*
> *3½ cups water*
> *2½ cups sugar*

1. Peel lemons, leaving peel as intact as possible while keeping the white pith to a minimum. Place lemon peels in 2-quart pitcher.
2. Pour vodka over lemon peels and place lid on pitcher or otherwise cover, sealing in mixture. Allow mixture to sit at room temperature for 4 days.
3. After 4 days, combine water and sugar in large saucepan and cook on medium for 5 minutes or until sugar is completely dissolved. Remove mixture from heat and allow to cool completely.
4. Add sugar mixture to vodka and lemon peels, cover pitcher again, and let stand overnight.
5. The next day, strain limoncello and throw away lemon peels. Pour mixture into vodka bottle with lid

or another lidded bottle. Refrigerate for at least 4 hours before serving.

MAKES: 20 servings

· · · · · · ·

JALAPEÑO MARGARITA

I love a spicy margarita to go along with all of those yummy taco recipes. This recipe is so delicious, I've made it multiple times and love it every time. And it took only once for me to realize that you need to use a fork when working with that jalapeño or you'll stick your jalapeño fingers in your eye and the party is OVER. I will also warn you that if you aren't a huge fan of the heat, just rim your glass with salt and skip the cayenne.

PREP TIME: 10 minutes

2 teaspoons fine sea salt
dash cayenne pepper
juice of 1 lime
ice
2 ounces tequila
1½ ounces Grand Marnier
4 slices jalapeño pepper
½ ounce simple syrup
lime wedge for garnish
jalapeño slices for garnish

1. Pour sea salt and cayenne pepper on small plate and mix.

2. Using lime juice, coat rim of rocks glass, then swirl glass on cayenne and salt plate. Fill with ice and set aside.

3. In cocktail shaker, add ice, tequila, Grand Marnier, jalapeño, and simple syrup. Shake well and pour into rocks glass.

4. Garnish with lime wedge and 3 to 4 jalapeño slices.

MAKES: 1 serving

• • • • • • •

RASPBERRY VODKA REFRESHER

The world's easiest summer cocktail that also has next to zero calories. I put this together when I was bartending in New York. It's fizzy, fruity, and boozy. A winning combination on a hot day!

PREP TIME: 5 minutes

> *crushed ice*
> *2 ounces Raspberry Stoli*
> *juice of 1 lime*
> *4 ounces seltzer*
> *raspberries for garnish*
> *lime wedge for garnish*

1. Fill Collins glass with crushed ice. Pour Raspberry Stoli over ice and add lime juice and seltzer. Stir once.

2. Serve with 2 to 3 raspberries dropped in glass and lime wedge.

MAKES: 1 serving

. . . .

THE PERFECT G&T

My brother is one of the owners of Frank in Austin, Texas, where they have an amazing gluten-free menu as well as one for the "norms," and an exceptional coffee bar and cocktail menu to boot. The first time I had juniper berries in my G&T, I knew I had to start mixing mine up that way as well. An exceptional tonic like Fever Tree or Q really seals the deal.

PREP TIME: 5 minutes

2 ounces gin
juice of ½ lime
4 ounces tonic
1 large block of ice
juniper berries for garnish (if available)
lime wedge for garnish

1. In rocks glass, combine gin, lime juice, and tonic. Drop in 1 large block of ice, or 2 or 3 smaller cubes and push down ice to mix.
2. Drop 4 or 5 juniper berries in the glass, and garnish with lime wedge.

MAKES: 1 serving

. . . .

LILLET BLANC MARTINI

This is another refreshing martini that offers a kick of flavor. I love using Lillet Blanc as a mixer. The

French wine cocktail is perfect for Bastille Day (or any other day, quite frankly).

PREP TIME: 7 minutes

> *ice*
> *1 ounce Lillet Blanc*
> *1 ounce vodka*
> *2 ounces grapefruit juice*
> *fresh ginger*

1. Fill cocktail shaker with ice. Pour in Lillet Blanc, vodka, and grapefruit juice, and shake until chilled.
2. Pour into chilled martini glass, and using microplane, shave fresh ginger over cocktail.

MAKES: 1 serving

·THANKS AND STUFF·

First things first: Thank *you*, reader, for reading. Even if you're only reading the thank-yous, well, you certainly got something out of it today, did you not? I so appreciate all of you gluten haters (and the people who love them) out there reading my blog, reading my books, and hanging out with me virtually and IRL. All of you GFFs are inspiring and I'm proud to be part of the crew. Thank you!!!!

For making *The Gluten-Free Cheat Sheet* happen, I have to give big props to Marian Lizzi at Perigee and all the other fab Perigee/Penguin people who are behind this super-fun project.

Of course, huge thanks go out to my fab agent, Alison Fargis, who always has the best ideas and guidance for gluten-free me. I also adore her office full of Stonesongers, who are amazing and always entertaining when I'm able to stop by and high-five everyone. You guys rock. Thanks for looking at videos of my kid on YouTube.

A huge thank-you and round of applause go to Maura Wall Hernandez, who developed some of the more amazing recipes in this here book. You can thank her for the Pumpkin Pound Cake, among others.

Thanks to my taste testers for plowing through these 100 recipes. Some of you thought you were coming over for dinner, but HA! Especially thanks to those of you who got the failures and wound up wondering if I had thought to make anything else for us to eat. No, I didn't. And I'm sorry.

To my gorgeous and genius support system, thanks one million times over: Catherine Crawford, Mac Montandon, Kara Dean and the boys, Victoria Harmer, Cary Fagan Whipple, Rebecca Coleman, Bart Coleman, the ladies of Las Vegas, Amy Slonaker for the freaking awesome pasta, the Mom.me and Whalerock team, the amazing folks at the WBT, Rebecca Dixon, Rebecca Woolf, Ellen Goldman, Amy Goldman, Sean Chandra, Swanhilda, Geoff Peveto, and the rest of the Peveto/Peveteaux/ Goldman/Reeves clan.

Thanks to my mom and dad for always thinking I was the "smart" one in the family. And of course, thanks to the three best roommates in the entire universe: Aaron, Esmé, and Judah—I adore you.

It's time to get out there and start experimenting. Taste, cook, and experience all that is to be had for you and your gluten-free loved ones so that you can find the joy in eating and socializing again. To help you get started on this journey, I've compiled a list of options, from my favorite mixes to my go-to chain restaurants, while also offering up sources for you to learn even more about how to survive and thrive while living gluten-free. Check out the blogs, and make some new gluten-free friends while you're at it! Please note that recipes, restaurants, and websites do change, and this information is the most up-to-date at the time of publication. Good luck and stay safe!

Support Groups

You're going to want to connect with other people in your same boat and talk about the ridiculousness of couscous at some point, so here are some great organizations that can help you out:

Celiac Disease Foundation (celiac.org)
National Foundation for Celiac Awareness
    (celiaccentral.org)
Raising Our Celiac Kids (celiackids.com)
Canadian Celiac Association (celiac.ca)
Celiac Sprue Association (csaceliacs.org)
National Institute of Health Celiac Disease
    Awareness Campaign (celiac.nih.gov)

Conferences and Expos

Celiac Disease Foundation National Conference (celiac.org). This annual conference and expo attracts the best in the industry, and I've personally been attending every year since receiving my celiac diagnosis. It takes place in the Los Angeles area every year, most recently making Pasadena its home base.

***Living Without*'s Gluten-Free Food Allergy Fest** (glutenfreefoodallergyfest.com). The *Living Without* magazine family has branched out to host gluten-free food festivals all around the country. With hundreds of exhibitors, bloggers, and G-free peeps, you will eat and meet well.

Gluten-Free and Allergen-Friendly Expo (gfafexpo .com). From California to Massachusetts with stop-offs in between, this is the largest gluten-free expo in the United States.

Food Allergy Bloggers Conference (fablogcon.com). Even if you're not a blogger, this is a fun festival held every year in Las Vegas with fantastic speakers and events.

There are also many local support groups, so check out your area meet-ups and offshoots of any of the organizations just mentioned and get out there!

Good Gluten-Free Reads

There are also some fantastic periodicals you can subscribe to or check out online to stay up-to-date on all of the latest gluten-free news, while enjoying new recipes and stories from people who are living gluten-free:

> *Gluten Free & More* (formerly *Living Without*) (livingwithout.com)
> *Allergic Living Magazine* (allergicliving.com)
> *Simply Gluten Free* (simplygluten-free.com)
> *Delight Gluten Free* (delightglutenfree.com)
> *Australian Gluten-Free Life* (agfl.com.au)
> *Gluten-Free Living* (glutenfreeliving.com)

MY FAVORITE GLUTEN-FREE COOKBOOKS AND GUIDES

> *Gluten Is My Bitch: Rants, Recipes, and Ridiculousness for the Gluten-Free* by . . . me! Why, yes, this is my book, and that's why I think you should have it. Especially if you're feeling

ranty or ridiculous or in need of some gluten-free chicken and waffles.

Gluten Freedom by Alessio Fasano, MD, with Susie Flaherty. The preeminent expert on celiac disease, treatment, and the future of gluten-free, Dr. Fasano explains it all to those of us living with the pain of not being able to eat croissants.

The Essential Gluten-Free Restaurant Guide by Triumph Dining. An excellent resource in print or online, these are the people who bring you the "I'm gluten-free" cards in every language.

Nosh on This: Gluten-Free Baking from a Jewish-American Kitchen by Lisa Stander Horel and Tim Horel. Lisa and Tim have perfected the texture of gluten-free breads and cookies. If you've been missing challah, they will show you the way.

1,000 Gluten-Free Recipes by Carol Fenster. A great place to start. Carol Fenster is one of the best gluten-free cookbook writers around. In fact, someone probably gave you this book the minute you said you were going gluten-free.

Gluten-Free on a Shoestring by Nicole Hunn. A solid cookbook filled with delicious recipes. Nicole Hunn's books are all worth picking up and digging into.

Artisanal Gluten-Free by Kelli Bronski and Peter Bronski. The first gluten-free cookbook I ever owned. The Bronskis make gluten-free gourmet. A great resource for when your dining routine gets a bit boring.

The How Can It Be Gluten-Free Cookbook by the editors at America's Test Kitchen. The experts at the Test Kitchen have perfected a variety of gluten-free breads and many other recipes. You can always trust a cookbook from America's Test Kitchen, and it's beyond exciting that they went gluten-free.

The Warm Kitchen by Amy Fothergill. A lovely lady and chef, Amy Fothergill creates easy, home-cooked meals that are truly from the heart.

Celiac and the Beast by Erica Dermer. A girl after my own sarcastic heart, Erica Dermer has written a laugh-out-loud tale of one girl's gluten challenges and the weird things that can happen when you're on the road to wellness-ish.

The Complete Guide to Living Well Gluten-Free by Beth Hillson. She's not joking when she calls this the "complete" guide. Buy this book and you'll use it as a reference tool for everything from picking a physician to getting over getting gluten-ed.

The Gluten-Free Table: The Lagasse Girls Share Their Favorite Meals by Jilly Lagasse and Jessie Lagasse Swanson. Yep, it's *those* Lagasse girls, and having a professional chef for a dad has absolutely helped these ladies out when they had to go G-free. In addition to creating mouthwatering gluten-free recipes, these sisters are adorable, and you can't help being charmed by them.

The Everyday Art of Gluten-Free by Karen Morgan. The lady behind Austin's Blackbird Bakery, Morgan has a way with pastry. You'll want this book if only for the "donut" flour blend.

Weeknight Gluten-Free by Kristine Kidd. An expert in the kitchen, Kidd has been doing the gluten-free cookbook thing for some time, and it shows. This book is essential when you want to get food on the table.

It Starts with Food: Discover the Whole30 and Change Your Life in Unexpected Ways by Dallas and Melissa Hartwig. I like to call the Whole30 "Paleo Extreme" because you're giving up everything you would on the Paleo diet and more! While it's not a great time, it has always helped my body heal if I've accidentally ingested gluten. I would recommend doing the Whole30 a month before any vacation you take just so you can start off feeling healthy and lose those few extra pounds before you slip on your bathing suit.

Vitamins and Medications

I prefer Country Life vitamins for all of my "Oh my God, I'm deficient!" needs. This brand is gluten-free and trustworthy. For any other drugs you're taking, whether they are vitamins, over-the-counter, or prescription, refer to Glutenfreedrugs.com and always, always, always talk to your physician about what you're ingesting as well.

Just Eat It

Now let's talk about food!

Before we break everything down by type, I'm going to give my four-star recommendations across the board. These brands are what I always have in my kitchen, whether it's for cooking or snacking.

APRIL'S ALL-STARS

Almond Milk LA almond milk
Bob's Red Mill almond meal
Cup 4 Cup all-purpose gluten-free flour
Dorot frozen herbs and garlic
Glutino table crackers
Justin's almond butter
Manischewitz gluten-free matzo
Primal Pasture organic, grass-fed meat
The Pure Pantry pancake mix
Scharffen Berger chocolate
So Delicious Dairy-Free Ice Cream (variety, but
    love the GF cookies and cream)
Trader Joe's gluten-free chicken, beef, and
    vegetable broth
Trader Joe's gluten-free corn pasta

Trader Joe's gluten-free hard shell tacos
Trader Joe's organic black beans
Udi's or Glutino sandwich bread
Weekly order from Good Earth Organics, CSA
Whole Foods gluten-free piecrust
Wright's Hickory Liquid Smoke (gluten-free and
   soy-free)
XO Baking Co. pancake mix

Yes, we do eat well in the Peveteaux home. It's incredibly important for me (see Chapter 4, "Depression, Anxiety, and General Crankiness") to know that I have the makings of a great-tasting and safe dinner right at my fingertips. So I keep our kitchen stocked. Sometimes overstocked, as you should see my freezer right now. These brands help make that happen.

Here are some other great gluten-free brands you should check out:

BREAKFAST CEREALS/TREATS

Arrowhead Mills Gluten-Free Steel Cut Oats
Bob's Red Mill Gluten-Free Muesli
Bob's Red Mill Granola
Bob's Red Mill Mighty Tasty Hot Cereal
Cocomama Quinoa Cereal
Cream of Rice
General Mills Rice and Corn Chex
Glutenfreeda Gluten-Free Oatmeal
Glutino Toaster Pastries
KIND Granola
Kinnikinnick Donuts
Nature's Path Amazon Flakes
Nature's Path Gorilla Munch

Nature's Path Gluten-Free Organic Whole O's
Nature's Path Koala Crisps
Nature's Path Peanut Butter Panda Puffs
Purely Elizabeth Granola
Udi's Granola

BREADS

Against the Grain French Bread
Brazi Bites Cheese Bread
Bread Srsly (sourdough)
Canyon Bakehouse Hamburger Buns
Canyon Bakehouse Sandwich Bread
Glutino English Muffins
Glutino Sandwich Bread (variety of types)
Rudi's Sandwich Bread
Schar Ciabatta
Schar Dinner Rolls
Udi's Sandwich Bread (variety of types)
Whole Foods gluten-free cheddar biscuits

Check your local gluten-free bakeries for gluten-free bread, cakes, and treats. Those will be fresh baked and delicious, and there are new options popping up all over town every day. Yes, even your town!

PASTA

Ancient Garden Organic Quinoa (variety of types)
Andean Dream Quinoa (variety of types)
Barilla (variety of types)
Bionaturae (variety of types)
DeBoles Corn (variety of types)

Ener-G Lasagna Noodles
Glutino (variety of types)
Jovial Brown Rice (variety of types)
Le Veneziane Corn (variety of types)
Lundberg Brown Rice (variety of types)
Manini's (variety of types)
Schar's (variety of types)
Trader Joe's Brown Rice (variety of types)
Trader Joe's Corn (variety of types)

CRACKERS

Breton GF Original with Flax
Crunchmaster Multi-Seed
Glutino Bagel Chips
Glutino Table Crackers
Manischewitz gluten-free matzo
Mediterranean Snacks Sea Salt Lentil Crackers
Schar Saltines Table Crackers
Skinny Crisps
Van's Say Cheese

CANDY BARS

Amy's
Andy's Dandy Candy Bars
Dove Chocolate Bars
Endangered Species Chocolates
Enjoy Life Ricemilk Crunch
Hershey's Chocolate Bar
Hershey's Chocolate Bar with Almonds
Justin's Peanut Butter Cups
Scharffen Berger Chocolate Bars

PIZZA

Against the Grain

Amy's

Glutino

Lou Malnati's GF pizza (mail-order or in-store only—Chicago, Illinois)

Udi's

BBQ SAUCE

Annie's

Bone Suckin' Sauce

Bullseye Original BBQ Sauce

Stubb's

ALL-PURPOSE GLUTEN-FREE FLOURS

Better Batter

Bob's Red Mill

Carol's

Cup 4 Cup

Hodgson Mill

Jules Gluten Free

King Arthur Flour

Namaste

Pamela's

XO Baking Co.

THIS IS HOW MANY DELICIOUS GF PANCAKE AND WAFFLE MIXES EXIST

Arrowhead Mills

Bisquick

Bob's Red Mill

Cherrybrook Kitchen

Cup 4 Cup

Glutino

Hodgson Mill

King Arthur

Maple Grove Farms

Namaste

Nicole's Naturals

Pamela's

The Pure Pantry

Stonewall Kitchen

XO Baking Co.

GLUTEN-FREE BEER

Brunehaut

Estrella Damm Daura (gluten removed)

Glutenator

Glutenberg IPA

Green's Dubbel Dark

Harvester IPA

Ipswich Celia Saison

New Grist

New Planet Pale Ale

Omission IPA (gluten removed)

Steadfast

St. Peter's Sorghum Beer

FOOD DELIVERY

Now that we've covered the individual food substitutions you'll want to seek out and experiment with, let's talk about getting gluten-free food delivered right to your door. There are two different ways this can happen: One is a meal delivery service, and the other is a monthly subscription box. They both serve the purpose of getting you to expand your gluten-free horizons. Here are a few services that deliver gluten-free goodness:

Freshology.com: This meal delivery service can feed you every meal, every day, if you'd like to never have to cook again. A chef and a nutritionist design gluten-free gourmet meals that are not only delicious but healthy, too.

WorldGardensCafé.com: This business caters to people looking to lose weight as well as those on specialty diets. You can subscribe monthly and receive all the premade meals at the beginning of each week, so you don't have to think about it again for 30 days.

PaleoDelivers.com: If you're in Southern California, these chefs make gluten-free and Paleo meals and snacks that come fresh to your door. In addition to being gluten-free, all the meals are sustainable and organic.

FoodFlo.com: Another SoCal chef, Flo provides vegan and gluten-free meals by the week with her program. As the mother of an autistic child, she recognized the effect food could have, and committed to vegan and gluten-free living. She also has specially designed "Flo-bars" for "pick me up" snacks.

Cookiesconamore.com: Just cookies, but oh, what cookies. Delicious Italian cookie favorites have gone gluten-free, and you can order boxes and boxes. Move over, Girl Scouts.

SUBSCRIPTION BOXES FOR GLUTEN-FREE FOOD

Find Me Gluten-Free/Send Me Gluten-Free: The fantastic app that helps the gluten-free diner find safe restaurants all over the world now has a subscription box. The attention to detail in the original endeavor makes me believe this is going to be a great one.

The Tasteful Pantry: This is another company that will create a box based on your various food requirements. This one is also well curated and a blast to open up each month. You can also order just a "treat box" if that's what you're in the mood for that month.

Love with Food: This monthly snack box can be customized on many levels. One of my favorites is when K.C. of G-Free Foodie curates an exceptional gourmet gluten-free box. But the most exciting thing about this subscription box is that for every box purchased, Love with Food donates a meal to a nonprofit organization that feeds the hungry.

CHAIN RESTAURANTS WITH GLUTEN-FREE MENUS

Abuelo's
B.J.'s Brewhouse
Bucca di Beppo
Buddha's Belly
California Pizza Kitchen
Carrabba's
Chuck E. Cheese
Claim Jumper
The Counter
Crust Pizza
Don Pablo's
El Pollo Loco
Fleming's
Fresh Brothers
Garlic Jim's
Jason's Deli
Logan's Roadhouse
Maggiano's
Maudie's Tex Mex
The Melting Pot
My Fit Foods
The Old Spaghetti Factory
Olive Garden
On the Border
Outback Steakhouse
Pei Wei
P.F. Chang's China Bistro
Pizza Rev
Red Robin
Romano's Macaroni Grill
ShopHouse Southeast Asian Kitchen

Texas Land and Cattle
True Food Kitchen
Uno Chicago Grill
Yard House
Z Pizza

BEST LOCAL GLUTEN-FREE BLOGS

I love using the Locate Special Diet and Find Me Gluten-Free apps when I travel. Not only can these be a lifesaver when you're in a new area, but it's also fantastic to peek inside the local gluten-free scene when you're out there on the road. It never hurts to e-mail gluten-free bloggers and ask for their favorite recommendations. And you just might make a gluten-free friend. Here are some great resources for local gluten-free restaurant recommendations around the USA:

Alabama: Glutenfreebirmingham.com is a guide for products, restaurants, and events as well as the personal challenges of being a gluten-free kid. RocketCity Mom.com is a parenting site, but this lady is gluten-free and has explored the neighborhood, which means her list of gluten-free restaurants is extensive for the Huntsville area.

Alaska: Allergyfreealaska.com has got you covered from Anchorage to Eagle River. Bookmark this site and start making your Alaska dream trip come true.

Arizona: CeliacandtheBeast.com can point you in the right direction around Phoenix and Tucson while dishing up the snark as well. Bonus! This girl travels and reviews gluten-free restaurants as she goes. TheCheeky

Celiac.com is also a traveler (check out her posts on Disneyland for your GF kids!), and she fills us in on gluten-free dining in the many resorts of Arizona.

Arkansas: If you're in northwest Arkansas or southwest Missouri, NWAFoodie.blogspot.com can hook you up. Her latest restaurant-recommendation post offers up info about chain restaurants as well, so you should be able to travel the state without fear.

California: Well, this is impossible because I know a ton of GF bloggers and resources in California, and I'm for sure going to leave one or five out. So here's the short list. SoCal—Glutenfreeinsb.wordpress.com (Santa Barbara), GlutenIsMyBitch.wordpress.com (that's me, and I'm in the LA area), and Glutenfreeinsd.com (San Diego). NoCal—Fearlessdining.com and GFinSF.com (San Francisco Bay area).

Colorado: Now that's what I call a database! Gigcolorado.org offers an extensive list of restaurants based on your address in Colorado. This support group is less blog and more "basic information I need right this minute." I have a feeling no gluten-free person goes hungry in the Centennial State.

Connecticut: Complete with an interactive map, Glutenbgone.wordpress.com covers all of Connecticut when talking gluten-free restaurants.

Delaware: I'm not sure if I should apologize to the people of Delaware for saying the best dining-out information can be found on the site Glutenfreephilly.com. Whether you search his website or download his guide to eating gluten-free in Philly and Delaware, this guy knows his gluten-free stuff all up and down the mid-Atlantic.

Florida: CeliacinOrlando.com not only gives local recommendations but also has a full section on navigating Disney World. Follow @gfinorlando on Instagram for tasty bites as well as recipes.

Georgia: Georgiarock.org is a site for celiac kids, and you know kids—they get hungry. Hence the extensive list of gluten-free restaurants as well as support for families.

Hawaii: When I was searching for local blogs that covered gluten-free Hawaii, I kept coming across gluten-free writers who travel to those beautiful islands. While this is great info, it's not as comprehensive as a local might publish. So enjoy the travel blogs, and check out CeliacRestaurantGuide.com and search the list for Hawaii.

Idaho: Donteatwheat.com is the story of a mother and daughter with gluten and dairy intolerances and a husband (a doctor) who is a mindful eater. In addition to their own food philosophy, which leans toward Paleo, they offer an extensive list of chain and local Idaho, Utah, and California restaurants that are gluten-free.

Illinois: Frannycakes.com offers up amazing recipes, a beautifully designed site, and tips on where to find gluten-free donuts in Chicago. You'll love her. You'll also love Glutenfreebetsy.com, which gives you all the gluten-free restaurant information you'll need if you're in the Chicago area. Yes, all.

Indiana: Glutenfree219 serves Indiana and the Chicago area with one of the most organized restaurant recommendation lists you'll ever lay eyes upon. Go forth to Indiana and eat safely, my gluten-free friends.

Iowa: While gluten-free restaurants in Iowa seem to be multiplying with every Google search, there aren't a lot of people blogging about gluten-free in the Hawkeye State. Since Iowagirleats.com was diagnosed with celiac this year, I would watch her blog for tips when you visit the area. She's already stocked up her amazing blog with gluten-free recipes. Let's see if she can help us out when she hits the town.

Kansas: Celiacwichita.blogspot.com is an incredibly funny college student reviewing restaurants around town. Farther north in Kansas City is Glutenfreeformen .com, but as a lady, I can tell you I enjoyed the recipes, reviews, and ode to gluten-free BBQ sauce very, very much.

Kentucky: Glutenfreelouisville.org and Glutenfreelex ington.org are both great sources for restaurants the gluten-free can enjoy safely. But really, all you need to know about gluten-free dining in Kentucky is that bourbon is gluten-free.

Louisiana: Follow @loringaudin on Instagram for scrumptious gluten-free restaurant recommendations and pics in New Orleans.

Maine: Eatdrinkbetter.com isn't strictly gluten-free, but it does have a gluten-free restaurant guide for Portland, Maine, and these restaurants sound delicious.

Maryland/Washington, DC: Citylifeeats.com is out on the town a lot, which makes it challenging to stay gluten-free. Lucky for us, she shares her hard-won knowledge about local restaurants. Glutenfreegimmethree.com is an irreverent gluten-free blogger who also gets out and about. She also lets us know when a restaurant is *not* safe, which is incredibly helpful as well.

Massachusetts: Glutenfreebostongirl.com covers Massachusetts dining far afield of Harvard Square. This college student dines out often while keeping safe and has created an extensive list for the rest of us.

Michigan: Glutenfreegimmethree.com is originally from Detroit, which means you can find some great gluten-free restaurant reviews in that area on her blog as well. Gfreemonkey.com is adorable, and she blogs about gluten-free-friendly restaurants around Grand Rapids, Holland, and wherever her travels take her.

Minnesota: Thesavvyceliac.com is a one-stop shop when you're learning about celiac disease. Amy also has a slew of restaurant recommendations all around Minnesota that sound divine.

Mississippi: Around the Jackson area (and beyond, as this girl travels), Glutenfreegirlms.com fills you in on the best GF options while dining out. Down south you can get restaurant recommendations from Glutenfree southmississippi.com.

Missouri: From Joplin to Branson, Glutenfreepearls .com lays all the gluten-free restaurants out on the line for you. And if St. Louis is your locale, Theceliaclady .blogspot.com has a list of go-to places to make your gluten-free belly full.

Montana: For the best gluten-free Missoula has to offer, Glutenfreemontana.blogspot.com will keep you up-to-date.

Nebraska: Lincolncelicas.org provides a list that is definitely chain-heavy but safe for the gluten-free. Follow @GlutenfreeOmaha on Twitter to get the latest on gluten-free dining in the area.

Nevada: Glutenfreelasvegas.weebly.com will set you up before you ever head out to the tables. Vegas is great for gluten-free, and you'll find a huge list of options here. If you're headed to Sparks or Reno, check out the "Gluten Free in Reno and Sparks Nevada" Facebook page for great tips and community.

New Hampshire: It seems like a lot of people take lovely gluten-free trips up to New Hampshire, so you can find reviews on a variety of travel sites. Celiac corner.com has a great piece about autumn in New England and eating gluten-free in New Hampshire. Start there.

New Jersey: Glutenfreedairyfreenj.blogspot.com likes to travel and post about the great restaurant finds that kill two food culprits with one stone. Myglutenfreenj .com has an extensive list around Jersey as well.

New Mexico: A fantastic list of gluten-free eats in Albuquerque and Santa Fe, Delectablyglutenfree.blogspot .com will guide you in the right direction. Luckily, the history of "clean" food in these areas means you will have a lot of options when you pass through these beautiful towns.

New York: Glutenfreeblondie.com gets out a lot in the big city and has fab recommendations to prove it. GlutenFreeways.com is actually an East Coast and West Coast blogger (he likes to move), so you can check out his recommendations on both sides of the country. Follow @nycgrubber on Instagram to discover the most amazingly delicious restaurants in New York City in full color.

North Carolina: Glutenfreeinnc.com is an exhaustive resource for those who eat gluten-free. Jeff covers the entire state himself, with the help of fantastic guest bloggers.

North Dakota: Try Urban Spoon and the apps for gluten-free dining in North Dakota.

Ohio: Glutenfreegang.org is also a chapter of the Gluten Intolerance Group of North America, which means it offers support with a side of support. A great resource not only for Central Ohio but also beyond, it's a fantastic place to start your Ohio research. Prettylittleceliac .com covers Columbus, Cincinnati, and Chicago while motivating you to work out.

Oklahoma: Start with Okceliac.com for restaurant listings and support in the Oklahoma City area. Tulsa area gluten-free eaters, check out Glutenfreeindie.blogspot.com for an extensive list of area restaurants.

Oregon: Oregon is one of the gluten-freest states in the USA, so you can probably just walk into any restaurant and give someone a look and they'll bring you a gluten-free meal. Still, if you want to research beforehand, check out Glutenfreeportland.org and Anniesgluten freegrub.blogspot.com since she moved from San Diego to Portland.

Pennsylvania: I've already sung Glutenfreephilly.com's praises, and you can't beat his site for the area surrounding Philadelphia. Outside the City of Brotherly Love, you should check out WhyCan'tWheatBeFriends .com. She is located in western Pennsylvania, close to Ohio, and you'll find local reviews. But her chain restaurant section is useful to those of us all over the United States.

Rhode Island: Clearly the gluten-free need to head to Rhode Island with the online group Glutenfreefriends ri.yolasite.com, which organizes regular outings to gluten-free-friendly restaurants. Luckily the group publishes its results on the blog, but you could shoot a note to the group leader before heading to Rhode Island to see if you could tag along some night.

South Carolina: What's better than vacationing in Charleston? Reading Glutenfreecharleston.com before you head to one of the most beautiful cities in the South.

It's got all the resources you need to eat well and be charmed by this gem of a city.

South Dakota: A food writer for the ArgusLeader.com (the local Sioux Falls paper) just happens to have celiac, and a daughter with celiac. This means great lists of gluten-free eats. Also, so inspirational!

Tennessee: Glutenfreegeek.com in Nashville has an interactive map so you can find out what gluten-free eats are closest to you while enjoying the Songwriting Capital of the World. If you're more of a Graceland fan, Ilovememphisblog.com has got you covered for gluten-free Memphis treats.

Texas: ATXglutenfree.com is also behind the Locate Special Diet app, so you know she's got Austin covered (and everywhere else—she spends a lot of time in Wyoming, too). GFreeinthecity.com is another great source of gluten-free eats in and around Austin. Lest you think I don't believe any other part of Texas exists, also check out DFWceliac.org for the Dallas–Fort Worth area and Houstonceliacs.org for good eats near the third coast.

Utah: The family from Idaho behind Donteatwheat.com also has recommendations in Utah for family- and gluten-free-friendly joints. Glutenfreeinutah.blogspot .com has fantastic links to bakeries, restaurants, and products found in Utah as well as other places she travels.

Vermont: So many great gluten-free products got their delicious start in Vermont that one would assume the

Green Mountain State would be an excellent place to go gluten-free. One would be right. Gfvermont.com has got you covered on all the latest gluten-free news up there.

Virginia: You can look to the fabulous group of gluten-free DC-area bloggers (as seen above) as well as Dcgluten-free.com for more lists of gluten-free eats around Virginia and the DC area. If you're not in that concentrated population, check out the Facebook page for Gluten-Free in Blacksburg, Virginia, for choices a bit farther out.

Washington: When you're married to a chef, you've got a line on all the good places, and Shauna of Glutenfreegirl.com is great about sharing their gluten-free gourmet finds. I also love Kathy at Gfreeandhappy .com for her infectious positivity and informative video series.

West Virginia: Load up your restaurant-finding apps when you head to West Virginia, but be sure to stop by (and check the blog) VenerableBean.blogspot.com in Morgantown. The gluten-free and vegan baked goods look amazing and can also be found at the Mountain Peoples Food Co-Op.

Wisconsin: Celiacinthecity.wordpress.com is based in Milwaukee, but CITC also reviews restaurants in other parts of the state, as she's quite the traveler. Search her site for #GlutenfreeinMKE for even more recommendations.

Wyoming: The Jackson Hole Dining Guide (jhdining guide.com) is all-inclusive, with listings for not only gluten-free but vegetarian and vegan as well. Lexies kitchen.com offers up grocery store lists as well as safe gluten-free dining in Cheyenne.

Page numbers followed by "n" indicate notes.

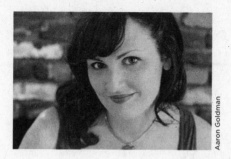

Aaron Goldman

April Peveteaux has been living with, and writing about, the gluten-free life since her celiac disease diagnosis in 2011. An editor and writer for parenting, lifestyle, and humor publications, she naturally turned her focus to the challenge of living gluten-free in a breadbasket-filled world once she was told "no more pie." Peveteaux is an advice columnist for *Gluten Free & More* by *Living Without*; an editor at Whalerock Industries' parenting site, Mom.me; and the author of the bestselling book *Gluten Is My Bitch: Rants, Recipes, and Ridiculousness for the Gluten-Free*. She lives and works in Los Angeles with her husband, two children, and pet fox.